the heart health guide

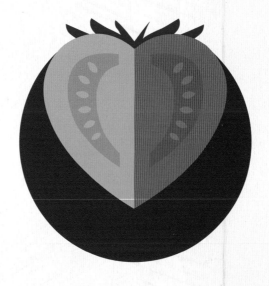

I dedicate this book to my mentors,
colleagues and research collaborators, and
my patients and study participants who
trusted in the scientific method and
volunteered to follow the Mediterranean
diet regimes to manage their condition and
provide evidence for future generations.

the heart health guide

DR CATHERINE ITSIOPOULOS (PHD APD)

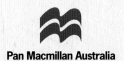

Pan Macmillan Australia

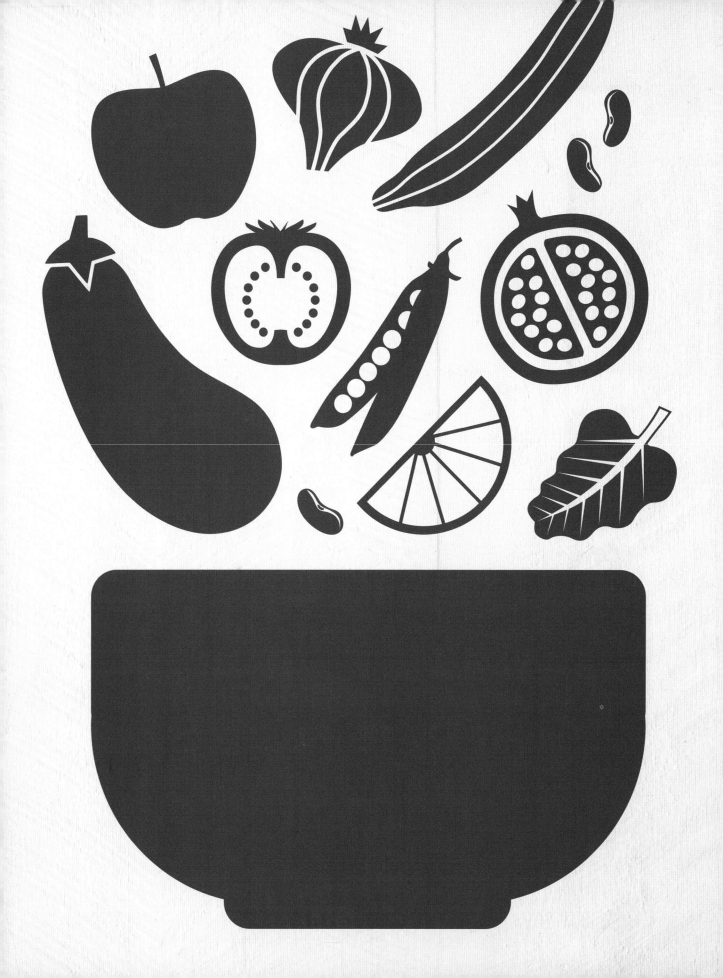

CONTENTS

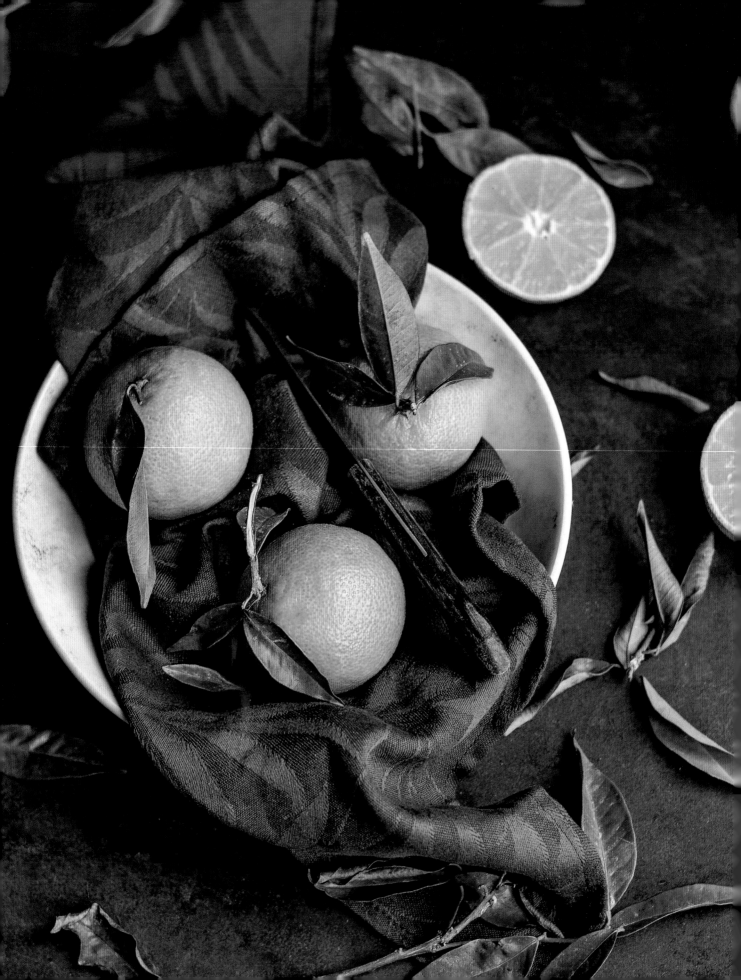

Introduction

As a clinical dietitian and nutritionist, my interest in the Mediterranean diet and lifestyle was sparked by the healthiness of Greek immigrants in Australia. Although I grew up in a Greek family who ate healthy Mediterranean cuisine, I came to understand the health benefits of this way of eating many years later as a clinical researcher. Compared with Australian-born people, they seemed relatively protected from chronic diseases such as heart disease – in fact, the risk of them developing this disease was 30 per cent lower than the average Aussie. This was due, in part, to their traditional Mediterranean diet and lifestyle habits.

I've now spent almost thirty years researching the health benefits of the Mediterranean diet on heart disease, diabetes, fatty liver, metabolic syndrome, asthma, dementia, depression and anxiety. Through my work, I have come to realise that this way of eating does wonders for tackling all of the chronic diseases that are related to poor diet and lifestyle habits. The breadth of plant-based ingredients and fermented dairy foods, seafoods and free-range animal foods included in this diet provides an optimal combination of nutrients that work in a unique, synergistic way to boost the body's antioxidant and anti-inflammatory defence systems and guard against diseases of the modern world.

When I first started researching the Mediterranean diet, there was very little in scientific literature about its health benefits or how it works. Today, there are almost 7000 scientific papers reported in the published literature, and more than 2500 of them are focused on investigating its impact on heart disease.

I have concentrated my research on heart disease because it remains the major killer in Australia and across the world: about 50 people per day die in Australia of heart disease, and in the US, one person every 40 seconds dies of heart disease. Incredibly, almost 90 per cent of heart disease deaths can be prevented by following healthy lifestyle habits such as not smoking, exercising daily and eating a plant-based diet rich in fruits and vegetables such as the Mediterranean diet.

Changing your diet and lifestyle can be hard, and it's easy to be tempted by fad diets that promise massive weight loss or miracle cures for diseases. My advice is that if something sounds too good to be true, then it just isn't true. Unlike the thousands of fad diets out there, the Mediterranean diet is a traditional eating pattern that dates back to antiquity and continues to be a way of living that keeps us healthy no matter how the world around us changes.

I am excited to present to you my third book on the Mediterranean diet. In creating this book I worked closely with my dearest research colleagues – leading experts in cardiology, metabolic diseases and dietetics who are profiled on page 234 – to bring together the current scientific evidence of this diet and to illustrate how it works to protect the heart. I also worked with my loving family, especially my daughters Vivienne and Tiana who love to cook and inspired many of the vegetarian and vegan-friendly dishes.

Part 1 will arm you with a deeper understanding of how this diet protects the heart from heart disease, Part 2 will provide you with a detailed analysis of the beneficial ingredients, and Part 3 is your toolkit on how to incorporate the diet into your everyday life for optimal heart health. In the final section you will find 80 delicious recipes for you to enjoy with your family and friends. I hope you embrace the Mediterranean way of life for heart health, happiness and longevity.

An ancient diet with modern benefits

Unlike most of the diets that crowd our modern landscape, the traditional Mediterranean diet dates back to ancient times (5000–2000 BC) with the key defining ingredients being wheat, wine and olive oil as well as wild edible leafy greens and legumes. In the 1500s, Christopher Columbus and other European explorers returning from voyages to South America introduced a broad range of colourful new ingredients including citrus fruits, tomatoes, chillies, eggplants and potatoes. These were incorporated into the Mediterranean diet.

In 1989, American physiologist Ancel Keys and his colleagues published 'The Seven Countries Study'. This was the first time the traditional Mediterranean diet had been described in scientific literature. This study investigated the link between diet and lifestyle behaviours and death from heart disease and all causes. They found that the group of participants from the island of Crete in Greece had almost no deaths from heart disease after 15 years of follow-up, and they believed that this was due to their plant-based, olive oil-rich diet. Since then, this archetypal Cretan Mediterranean diet has been studied in relation to all types of health outcomes, and research continues to uncover the beneficial properties associated with the Mediterranean diet.

Though there are several countries besides Greece whose diets can be classified as being Mediterranean, and specifically 'Southern Mediterranean' – Greece, Cyprus, Spain, Portugal, Italy, Morocco – in this book, I'll be exploring the Cretan (or Greek) version of the Mediterranean diet, which is the diet I have been researching for much of my career.

WHY EXPERTS CONTINUE TO BE EXCITED BY THIS DIET

Research has consistently found that following a Mediterranean diet can protect from deaths caused by heart disease, stroke, type 2 diabetes, certain cancers, neurodegenerative diseases, Alzheimer's and other dementias – even in non-Mediterranean populations, including Australians. These results came from a review of past peer-reviewed research trials that investigated 37 different health outcomes in more than 12.8 million people around the world.

These trials found that for every point increase in the score of adherence to a Mediterranean diet (0 being no adherence and 9 being total adherence) there was a 10 per cent reduction in risk of death from heart disease, cancer (breast and prostate cancers in particular), Alzheimer's disease and other forms of dementia, neurodegenerative diseases such as Parkinson's disease, diabetes, stroke and death from any cause.

The Mediterranean diet has also been reviewed as the easiest dietary pattern to follow, the best plant-based diet, and best diet for healthy eating and diabetes management. Managing diabetes is important because it is a key risk factor for heart disease. A study I conducted with colleagues in Australia examined the impact of a diet modelled on the Cretan Mediterranean diet on the management of type 2 diabetes. This study showed that by incorporating the 10 key principles of the diet into their eating plans, study participants achieved better control of their blood sugar levels that was equivalent to drug therapy.

A panel of medical experts, dietitians and other health professionals who convened to rank the healthiest diet in the world recently found the Mediterranean diet to be the healthiest diet in

The Mediterranean diet ranked as the easiest diet to follow, the best diet for healthy eating, the best diet for diabetes and best diet overall.

the world for the third year running when compared with 41 other diets. Each diet is measured according to:

- the likelihood of short- and long-term weight loss while following it;

- its effectiveness against combatting and preventing heart disease, stroke and diabetes; and

- how easy it is to follow.

The Mediterranean diet ranked highest in 2018, 2019 and again in 2020 as the easiest diet to follow, the best diet for healthy eating, the best diet for diabetes *and* best diet overall!

A diet that's good for our planet

Increasingly, the health of our planet is talked about as something that goes hand in hand with the health of humans. The types of foods we eat and how they are grown play a role in the food system and determine the impact on the health of the planet. The World Health Organization (WHO) is encouraging a plant-rich diet that has a low environmental impact through lower resource use and greenhouse gas emissions.

The Mediterranean diet is a health-promoting and environmentally sustainable way to eat. When compared with a Western-style diet, the Mediterranean diet includes less meat and animal products – both of which use more land and water and produce more greenhouse gasses than plants. Experts estimate that by switching from a Western-style diet to a Mediterranean one, we could reduce greenhouse gas emissions by up to 72 per cent, land use by up to 58 per cent, energy consumption by up to 52 per cent, and water consumption by up to 33 per cent.

A recently commissioned international collaboration called the EAT-Lancet Commission pulled together experts from fields of human health, agriculture, political sciences and environmental sustainability from 16 countries across the world in order to develop global scientific targets for a sustainable, healthy diet and food production system capable of feeding up to 10 billion people by 2050.

This collaboration identified a universal healthy reference diet, which consists of fresh vegetables, fruits, wholegrains, legumes, nuts, and unsaturated oils, includes a low to moderate amount of seafood and poultry, and includes no (or a low quantity of) red meat, processed meat, added sugar, refined grains and starchy vegetables. The traditional Mediterranean diet as characterised by Ancel Keys is called out as an example of an eating pattern that meets these universal guidelines. Furthermore, the experts identify factors such as reducing food waste by at least 50 per cent and producing food sustainably as key to food security for the future.

In acknowledgement of the impact this diet and lifestyle pattern has had in Mediterranean populations over many centuries, it was inscribed on the UNESCO Representative List of the Intangible Cultural Heritage of Humanity in 2013. It is described by this UNESCO nomination as 'a diet and lifestyle pattern that involves a set of skills, knowledge, rituals, symbols and traditions concerning crops, harvesting, fishing, animal husbandry, conservation, processing, cooking, and particularly the sharing and consumption of food.' Women are called out as being the purveyors of this dietary pattern – the ones responsible for transmitting the knowledge and practices.

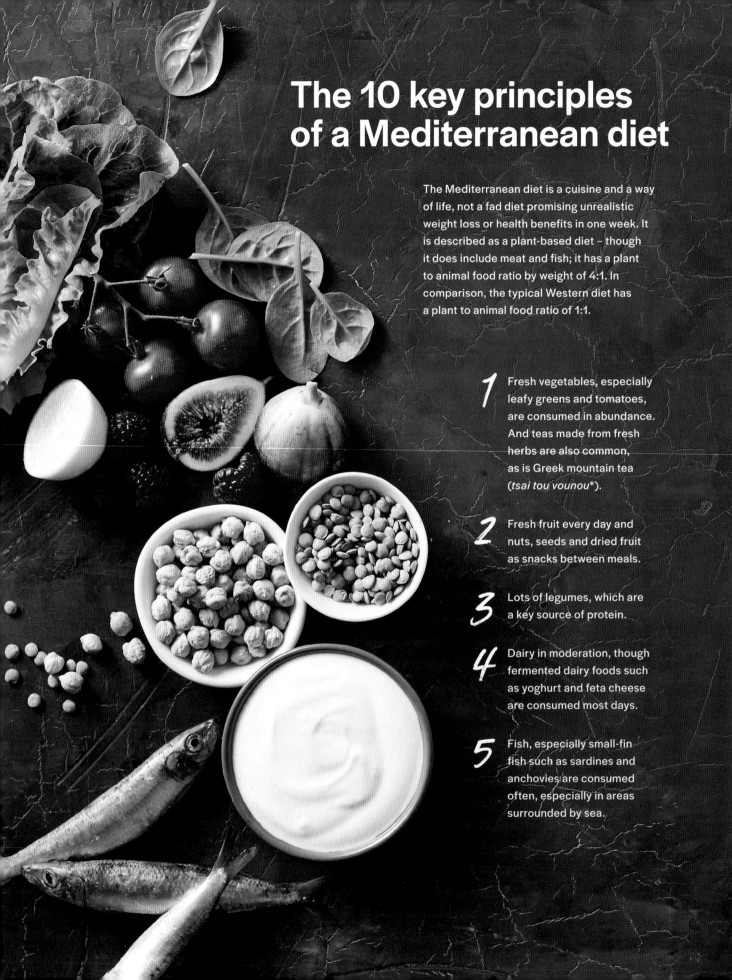

The 10 key principles of a Mediterranean diet

The Mediterranean diet is a cuisine and a way of life, not a fad diet promising unrealistic weight loss or health benefits in one week. It is described as a plant-based diet – though it does include meat and fish; it has a plant to animal food ratio by weight of 4:1. In comparison, the typical Western diet has a plant to animal food ratio of 1:1.

1 Fresh vegetables, especially leafy greens and tomatoes, are consumed in abundance. And teas made from fresh herbs are also common, as is Greek mountain tea (*tsai tou vounou**).

2 Fresh fruit every day and nuts, seeds and dried fruit as snacks between meals.

3 Lots of legumes, which are a key source of protein.

4 Dairy in moderation, though fermented dairy foods such as yoghurt and feta cheese are consumed most days.

5 Fish, especially small-fin fish such as sardines and anchovies are consumed often, especially in areas surrounded by sea.

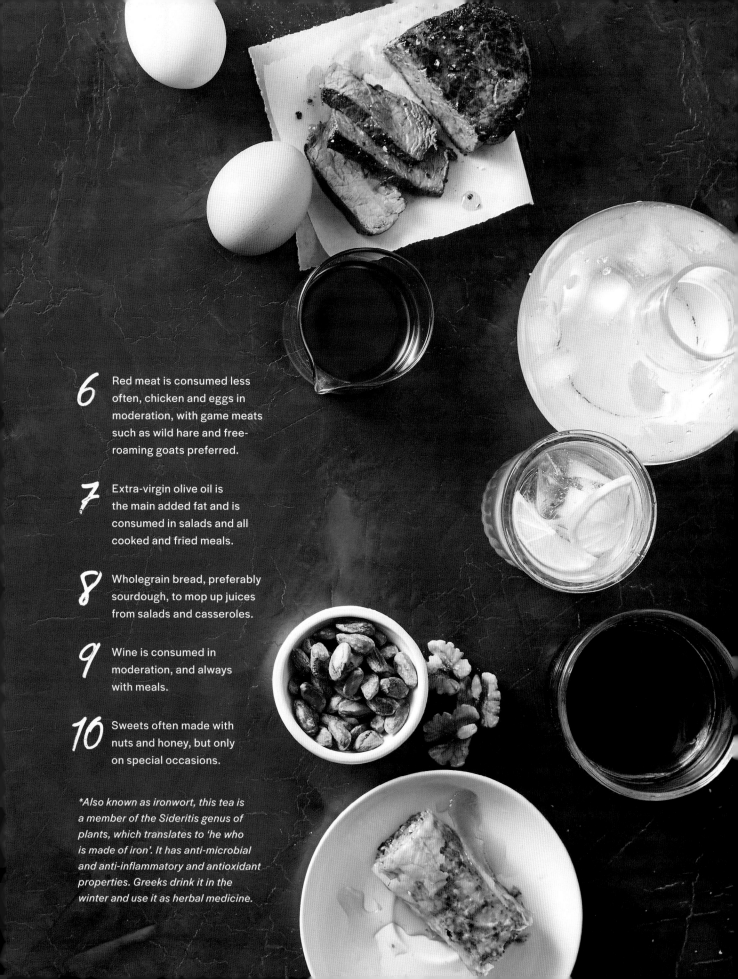

6 Red meat is consumed less often, chicken and eggs in moderation, with game meats such as wild hare and free-roaming goats preferred.

7 Extra-virgin olive oil is the main added fat and is consumed in salads and all cooked and fried meals.

8 Wholegrain bread, preferably sourdough, to mop up juices from salads and casseroles.

9 Wine is consumed in moderation, and always with meals.

10 Sweets often made with nuts and honey, but only on special occasions.

Also known as ironwort, this tea is a member of the Sideritis genus of plants, which translates to 'he who is made of iron'. It has anti-microbial and anti-inflammatory and antioxidant properties. Greeks drink it in the winter and use it as herbal medicine.

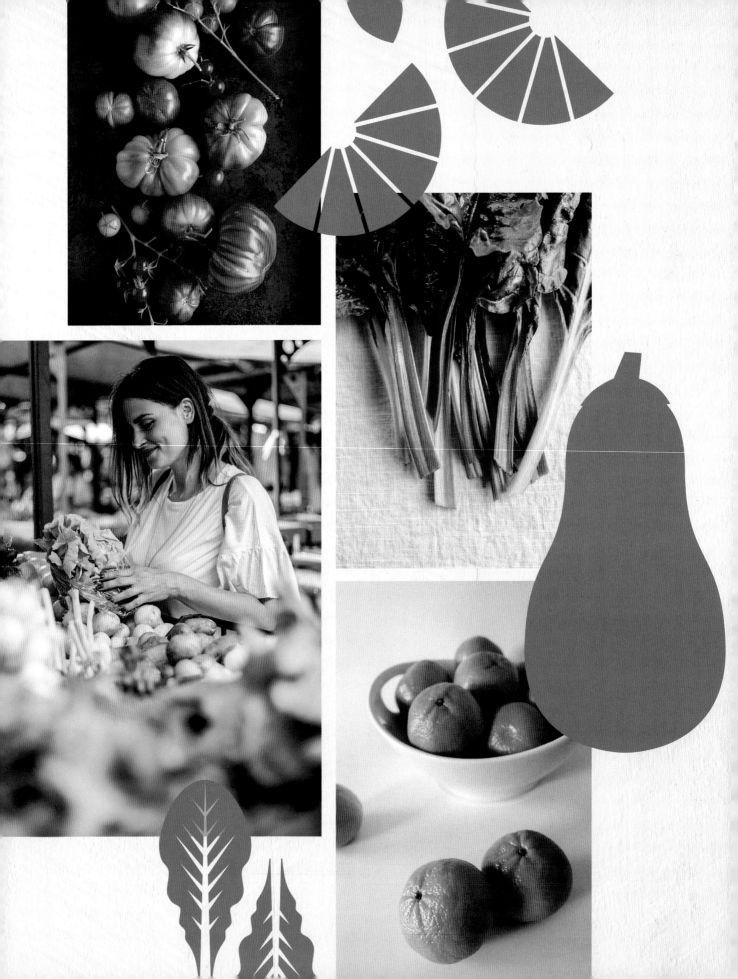

PART 1

Understanding *heart disease* and how it relates to diet

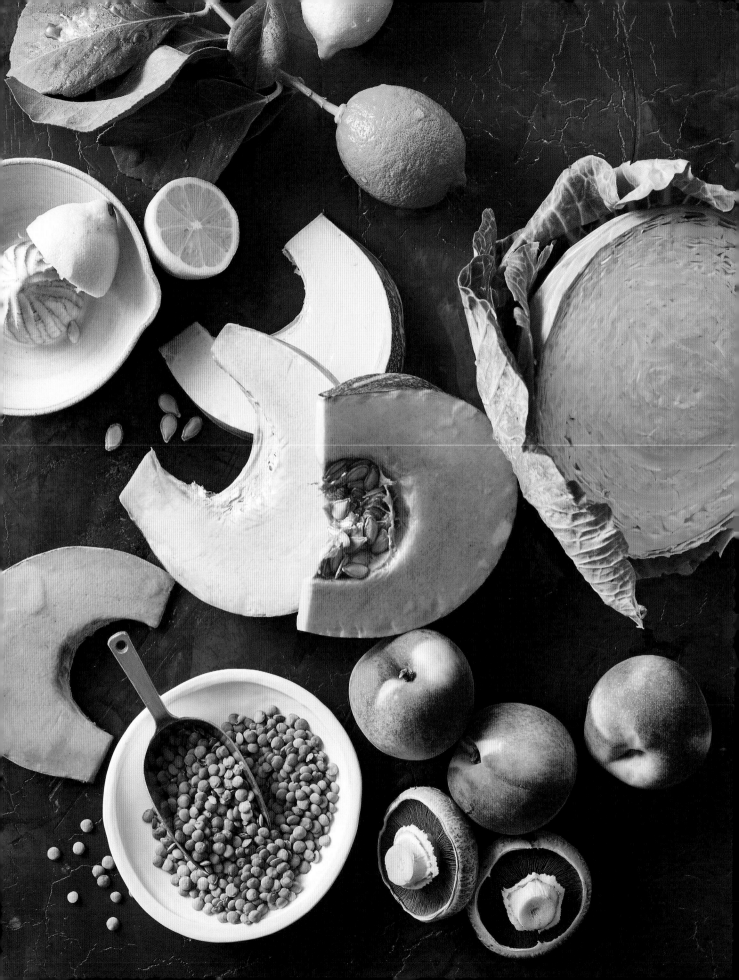

Heart disease:
A preventable assassin

Cardiovascular disease (CVD) is the collective term for diseases that affect the heart and blood vessels, such as stroke and coronary heart disease (also called heart disease). This family of diseases shares common risk factors such as poor diet and lifestyle. Heart disease is the most common cardiovascular disease and it remains the main cause of death in Australia and the world.

Your heart is the most important muscle in your body. Its main job is to pump oxygen-rich blood to every cell of the body. The heart is dependent on blood supply via the arteries that encircle it – the coronary arteries. The progressive narrowing of these coronary arteries is what causes heart disease. This narrowing is known as atherosclerosis and it occurs when 'plaque' builds up on the artery walls, causing the arteries to stiffen and narrow, in turn interrupting the blood supply to the heart.

Atherosclerosis can occur in any blood vessel in the body. When it occurs in the blood vessels that supply vital organs, such as the brain or the kidneys, it can lead to stroke or kidney failure (renal disease), respectively. And when plaque ruptures and oozes into the bloodstream, blood clots form and cause a complete blockage (or occlusion) in the coronary artery, stopping blood supply to the heart muscle. This leads to a heart attack or an infarction (also called myocardial infarction) and can be life threatening.

Historically, atherosclerosis (and heart disease) was thought to be caused solely by an increase in blood cholesterol accumulating in the artery walls leading to narrowing and, ultimately, a blockage and heart attack. Now it is well known that atherosclerosis begins when damage is done to the wall of the blood vessel through any number of risk factors such as smoking, high blood pressure, excessive alcohol intake, poor diet, obesity, type 2 diabetes or an imbalance in the gut microbiome. But it's not the damage itself that causes atherosclerosis, but rather the inflammation that occurs after the damage. Normally, inflammation is a process of repair: white blood cells are released and travel to the wound site to help fight infection. But in atherosclerosis, this low-grade inflammation causes white blood cells to attack the artery wall, called the endothelium, releasing inflammatory molecules. The artery wall is weakened and there's an accumulation of oxidised LDL (low density lipoprotein) or 'bad cholesterol', which has been chemically modified by free radicals. This oxidised LDL leads to plaque formation.

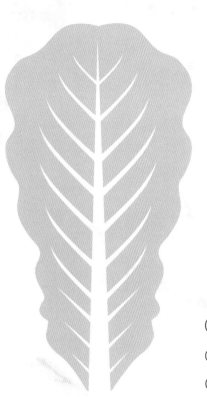

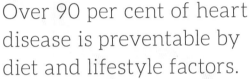

Over 90 per cent of heart disease is preventable by diet and lifestyle factors.

Heart disease continues to be the major cause of death across the world and a major threat to healthy longevity. It is estimated that over nine million people worldwide die of heart disease (ischaemic heart disease) each year; this and cardiovascular disease, which includes heart disease and stroke, remain the leading causes of death, accounting for one-third of all deaths.

About 50 people in Australia die each day of heart disease; in the US there is one death from heart disease every 40 seconds. Underlying risk factors such as obesity and diabetes continue to rise despite major public health efforts to improve these chronic diseases. Advancements in medical care, medications and heart surgery have significantly improved the survival of patients that have had a heart attack, however, these treatments come at a very high cost to the individual and the community, so we need a stronger focus on prevention.

Medical guidelines for the prevention and management of heart disease tend to focus on diet and other lifestyle behaviours as the first line of therapy for preventing that first heart attack and/or reducing a patient's risk of further heart attacks. Over the past decade, the focus has shifted away from individual nutrients such as fats or carbohydrate in favour on focusing on overall dietary patterns.

A comprehensive case control analysis across 52 countries comparing almost 30,000 people with and without heart disease included an evaluation of the links between diet, lifestyle and socioeconomic factors and the risk of having a heart attack. This study concluded that over 90 per cent of heart disease is preventable by diet and lifestyle factors, such as:

- **increasing fruit and vegetable intake;**

- **regular physical activity;**

- **moderate intake of alcohol; and**

- **not smoking.**

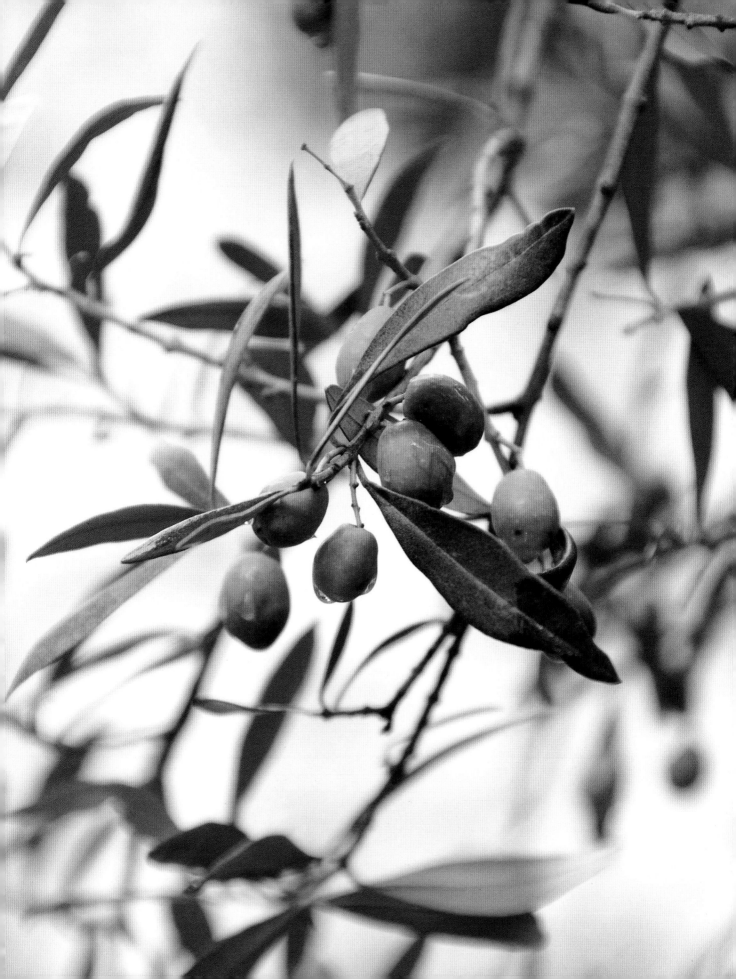

How cardiologists help patients reduce risk factors

Interview with DR ANDREW WILSON

Cardiovascular disease, or heart disease, is the number one cause of death in our community. The term cardiovascular disease includes heart attacks and strokes. People are more likely to have heart disease if they smoke, or if they have diabetes, high blood pressure or high cholesterol, or if people in their family have had heart disease. People who are inactive or overweight also have more risk of heart disease. Anything that improves these risk factors will reduce the risk of heart disease. Studies of the Mediterranean diet have shown that adherence to this diet improves many of these risk factors for heart disease and can prevent patients having heart disease.

Patients are often given medication to improve their risk of heart disease as well as advice on how to follow a healthy lifestyle, but that can be a lot of information to digest and they are often very stressed when they are diagnosed. Even so, talking about lifestyle and diet is a good step and can often give patients a positive direction in this stressful time.

Many patients are really interested to find out how they can improve their diet and activity when they know they have heart disease, and it is important that cardiologists understand how to give the right advice. Talking to my patients about the Mediterranean diet is often a positive thing as they like the idea of the food and I can tell them about how it improves heart disease risk. The patients that have started the diet really like it.

In addition to recommending patients avoid simple sugars (glucose, fructose, galactose and the like), I also talk to them about fibre. This is important for gut health, and fibre is a key part of the Mediterranean diet thanks to the diet's high levels of vegetables, grains and legumes. I discuss ways of cooking these ingredients with my patients. Different types of fibre feed our gut microorganisms and help maintain a healthy balance of bacteria in our gut. A healthy gut is associated with reduction in bowel diseases but also a reduction in fatty liver, inflammatory and allergic conditions such as asthma and arthritis.

Dr Andrew Wilson is an Associate Professor in the Departments of Cardiology and University Department of Medicine at St Vincent's Hospital and the St Vincent's Institute

Interview with DR MARNO RYAN

Diet quality has been directly linked to the risk of developing type 2 diabetes, which is a key risk factor for developing heart disease. The Mediterranean diet has been shown to reduce the risk of developing type 2 diabetes, as well as improve lipid profile and reducing systemic inflammation. Improvement in all these conditions leads to a reduction in fatty liver disease and cardiovascular disease.

Fatty liver, or non-alcoholic fatty liver disease (NAFLD), is closely associated with type 2 diabetes, obesity and cardiovascular risk. The Mediterranean diet has been demonstrated to reduce the degree of fat in the liver after only four weeks. A reduction in liver fat leads to a reduced risk of progression to chronic liver disease.

I like to talk to my patients with NAFLD and type 2 diabetes about the Mediterranean diet as it is something positive they can do to improve their conditions. Studies have demonstrated that people with a Mediterranean background are more likely to adhere more closely to this diet – presumably because they are already familiar with the ingredients that form the key elements of the diet.

For patients from a different dietary background, incorporating key elements of the Mediterranean diet into their daily routine is important. Identifying macronutrients in a particular ethnic cuisine and swapping them for the Mediterranean version is key. For example, suggesting that they use olive oil as the main added fat rather than the oil or fat they usually cook with, or highlighting fish as an important protein and source of unsaturated fat. These ingredients can then be incorporated into food eaten by different ethnic groups.

For patients for whom being overweight or obese is an issue, I emphasise an adequate intake of protein and fibre, as these macronutrients promote satiety – keeping them feeling fuller for longer. I also recommend they completely avoid simple sugars.

Exercising for at least 30 minutes a day is also crucial; this may simply be a walk, or a routine with light weights. Lifting weights in particular protects muscle, which is a vital component of metabolic rate, strength, mobility and quality of life.

Dr Marno Ryan is a gastroenterologist at St Vincent's Hospital

The research is positive

The most remarkable evidence in support of the cardioprotective effects of a Mediterranean diet is from a large Spanish study: The *Prevencion con Dieta Mediterranea Study* (PREDIMED), which tracked the health outcomes of nearly 7500 participants with risk factors for heart disease over a period of five years. These participants, whose risk factors included obesity and high blood pressure, were advised to follow a Mediterranean diet supplemented with 30 g nuts (walnuts, almonds, hazelnuts) per day or 1 litre of extra-virgin olive oil per week or a standard low-fat diet. At the end of the study, the people who followed a Mediterranean diet had a 30 per cent lower chance of dying from heart disease than those who followed the standard low-fat diet.

WHAT ABOUT POPULATIONS OUTSIDE THE SOUTHERN MEDITERRANEAN?

The Healthy Ageing Study (HALE) followed more than 2500 elderly Europeans from across that continent, including Scandinavian countries. It has found that closer adherence to a healthy lifestyle including combinations of non-smoking, moderate alcohol consumption, physical activity and adherence to a Mediterranean diet is associated with a more than 50 per cent lower risk of death from all causes, including heart disease.

In Melbourne, recent results from a large cohort study of over 42,000 healthy people who were followed for almost 15 years found that exercise and adherence to a Mediterranean diet were jointly associated with a 20 per cent reduction in the risk of dying from any cause. These results demonstrate that this dietary pattern can be effective in countries outside the Mediterranean.

The power of a Mediterranean diet to prevent a second heart attack in people that have already had a heart attack was elegantly demonstrated by the well-known Lyon Diet Heart Study by French clinical epidemiologist Professor Michel

Science versus social media

When assessing the weight of evidence of a link between a cause (e.g. diet or lifestyle factor) and an effect (a health issue such as heart disease), it is important to evaluate consistency. One study alone does not prove a theory, and many of the magical cures we read about or see in social media are reported by non-experts and based on anecdotes and testimonials. In the scientific community, the highest level of evidence is a systematic review and meta-analysis of well-controlled and expertly conducted studies from across the world. It's worth keeping this in mind next time an ad for the latest weight-loss miracle pops up in your feed.

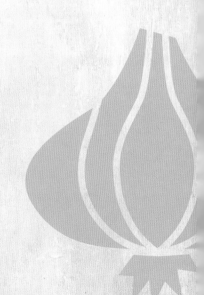

de Lorgeril and his colleagues in France in the late 1990s. In that study, about 800 people who had experienced a heart attack were randomly assigned a Cretan Mediterranean-style diet or standard low-fat diet, which they followed for four years. Remarkably, the study was stopped at the two-year mark by the ethics committee as the effects of a Mediterranean diet clearly outweighed the standard low-fat diet with a 70 per cent reduced risk of having a second heart attack in those following a Mediterranean diet.

This study has not been repeated over the past two decades, but my colleagues and I are continuing it and will be gathering data from multiple hospitals across the country. Our study is called the AUSMED Heart Trial and it follows the design of the Lyon Diet Heart Study. We plan to recruit more than 1000 people who have experienced a heart attack and randomly allocate them to a Mediterranean diet supplemented with nuts and extra-virgin olive oil or a standard low-fat diet to determine whether the Mediterranean diet can reduce the risk of having a second heart attack after 12 months. To date, we have studied just over 70 patients and have measured important changes in risk factors and markers of inflammation, which supports the claim that a Mediterranean diet has protective effects in people with heart disease.

Risk factor 1: Gut dysbiosis

Inflammation is the complex biological response of the body's tissues to infection and injury. In the first instance, our immune defence system neutralises threats such as viruses and infections by activating molecules that promote inflammation and destroy the threats. Once their job is done, inflammation-resolving molecules are activated to clear the damaged tissue components so that the body can begin to heal. However, if the immune system is repeatedly activated due to threats and is not allowed to heal properly, a persistent (or chronic) low-grade inflammation occurs.

We now know that inflammatory processes underlie many diseases, including heart disease. Systemic inflammation may be 'inflaming' the brain, vessels, joints and many organs, affecting their function and potentially contributing to the development of many chronic conditions including atherosclerosis, hypertension, diabetes, fatty liver, obesity, cancer, autoimmune conditions, osteoporosis, arthritis, inflammatory bowel diseases, kidney disease, dementia and depression. More research is needed, but it is agreed that 'low-grade systemic inflammation' is now considered to be the precursor to most chronic diseases.

Low-grade systemic inflammation is now considered to be the precursor to most chronic diseases.

Reducing inflammation has emerged as an important target for therapies in preventing or treating coronary heart disease.

Interestingly, the Mediterranean diet – compared to all other healthy diets – has been found to be protective against all the conditions mentioned on the previous page, leading many scientists to hypothesise that the Mediterranean diet benefits may be mainly due to its ability to reduce systemic inflammation. These conditions have also been linked to a disturbed gut microbiome.

Inflammatory cells release inflammatory chemicals that destabilise the fibrous cap covering the plaque, releasing its contents into the bloodstream of the coronary artery lumen (inside the tube of the artery). When plaques rupture, their components block blood supply to the heart, resulting in a heart attack.

Thanks to recent advances in imaging technologies it is now possible for us to see inflammatory cells inside blood vessels; they have been identified in greater numbers in patients who have damaged heart tissue following a heart attack. Consequently, reducing inflammation has emerged as an important target for therapies in preventing or treating coronary heart disease.

THE GUT MICROBIOME AND INFLAMMATION

Bacteria live in a variety of different locations in the human body including the gut, which is home to trillions of microorganisms. In fact, the colon is one of the most densely populated bacterial habitats on earth. The study of gut-dwelling bacteria is one of the most rapidly moving fields in research today thanks to promising interventions that focus on the health of the gut microbiome (all the microbes living in the gut) in order to maintain health and quality of life.

The microbes living in the gut offer many health benefits by participating in digestion and absorbing nutrients. Importantly, they also play a significant role in maintaining a barrier between the contents in the gastrointestinal tract and the body and participating in immune responses to kill harmful bacteria.

When a healthy microbiota is disrupted, it results in an imbalance between protective and harmful bacteria – this is known as dysbiosis. This condition is often characterised by reduced microbial diversity. Fewer beneficial bacteria mean the barrier between the gut and the body is harder to maintain, resulting in a 'leaky' gut that allows undesirable bacteria to migrate from the intestinal environment to the bloodstream, promoting inflammation.

Emerging research is pointing to a disturbed or 'dysbiotic' gut microbiome being the primary source of inflammation. Additionally, gut dysbiosis can also contribute to the development of obesity and insulin resistance, which are both important contributors to cardiovascular disease and type 2 diabetes. Given this, it's easy to see why maintaining a diverse and healthy gut microbiome is emerging as a strategy for promoting health, and preventing and managing disease.

Though genetics plays a role in gut microbiota, diet strongly influences gut microbial community structure and function. A healthy diet rich in plants sustains a healthy gut environment, but an unhealthy diet low in fibre with excess processed foods is likely to affect microbiota functional capability and contribute to disease susceptibility.

How inflammation and gut dysbiosis affect the body

A

Nervous
Parkinson's disease, Alzheimer's disease, other dementias

Musculoskeletal
Sarcopenia, osteoporosis, osteoarthritis, rheumatoid arthritis

Cardiometabolic
Cardiovascular disease, stroke, heart failure, diabetes

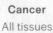

Pulmonary
Chronic obstructive pulmonary disease, bronchitis, emphysema

Cancer
All tissues

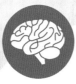

Digestive
Inflammatory bowel disease/colitis

B

Nervous
Parkinson's disease, Alzheimer's disease, multiple sclerosis

Musculoskeletal
Frailty, osteoporosis, rheumatoid arthritis, gout

Cardiometabolic
Obesity, diabetes

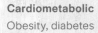

Pulmonary
Cystic fibrosis

Cancer
Colon

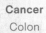

Digestive
Irritable bowel syndrome, Crohn's disease

TACKLING INFLAMMATION THROUGH A MEDITERRANEAN DIET

The Lyon Diet Heart Study discussed on pages 20–21 demonstrated that in people who had experienced a heart attack, following a Mediterranean diet reduced their risk of experiencing a second heart attack by 70 per cent compared with standard care (the usual prescribed treatment for heart disease being a low-fat diet). Interestingly, this dramatic effect was in spite of the diet having no significant impact on cholesterol levels, which were previously thought to have played a significant role in causing heart attacks. The protective effect was unlikely to be due to changes in blood fats such as cholesterol but more likely to be due to inhibition of inflammation by the anti-inflammatory effects of the foods and ingredients in the Mediterranean diet.

A large number of studies across the world have investigated whether putting people on a Mediterranean diet intervention has anti-inflammatory effects. Some of these studies have shown that following a Mediterranean diet leads to pronounced decreases in the presence of inflammatory markers in the blood and improves functioning of the lining of blood vessel walls more so than other diets.

The anti-inflammatory effects of a Mediterranean diet are promising not only for preventing development of coronary heart disease but also as a treatment method. Preliminary results from an ongoing trial in Spain of 1000 people who already have established coronary heart disease showed that a Mediterranean diet rich in extra-virgin olive oil improved levels of inflammatory markers. This diet also improved vascular function in a sub-group of those participants who also had type 2 diabetes.

What makes the Mediterranean diet anti-inflammatory?

In short: polyphenols. These bioactive compounds are found only in food and drinks sourced from plants, and many of them have proven antioxidant and anti-inflammatory properties. Research has shown that an increased polyphenol intake enhances the anti-inflammatory effect of following a Mediterranean diet.

The Mediterranean diet is rich in polyphenols thanks to fruit, vegetables, herbs and spices, wholegrains, nuts, seeds and legumes. Evidence suggests that consuming a variety of polyphenols increases the growth of beneficial gut bacteria thereby reducing inflammatory markers in the blood. Extra-virgin olive oil and red wine (which aren't typically included in other types of diet) also contain the polyphenols hydroxytyrosol, tyrosol, oleocanthal and resveratrol believed to have anti-inflammatory properties.

Extra-virgin olive oil has a higher polyphenol content than refined or light olive oil varieties, so consuming it is important to get the greatest anti-inflammatory effect.

A Mediterranean diet is also high in omega-3 fatty acids, largely from fish and also plant-based sources such as walnuts and certain wild leafy greens, which are associated with lower levels of inflammation in the body. Conversely, it also includes very low amounts of processed foods, high sugar drinks and red meat – the foods that promote inflammation.

The Mediterranean diet is high in both prebiotics (found in legumes and wholegrains) and probiotics (found in yoghurt and feta) – both of which are critical to maintaining a healthy and balanced microbiome. We'll explore these in detail and highlight the specific foods that provide these on page 39.

Risk factor 2: Dietary fats

Fat is often the first part of the diet that people think about when talking about heart disease. In the past, a low-fat diet was recommended for people with heart disease, but research now shows us that it is the type of fats consumed that are the most important.

Fat in food comes in many forms; it helps provide taste and a feeling of fullness, both of which allow us to enjoy eating. The good news is that the Mediterranean diet provides a moderately high amount of fat with much of it coming from beneficial monounsaturated fats and unsaturated omega-3 fats. These 'healthy' fats are eaten instead of less healthy fats, such as saturated and trans fats, which contribute to heart disease.

MONOUNSATURATED AND POLYUNSATURATED (OMEGA-3) FATS

More than half the fat in a Mediterranean diet comes from monounsaturated fats with the main source being extra-virgin olive oil. Other sources include avocados, peanuts and many tree nuts (almonds, hazelnuts). Monounsaturated fats help boost HDL 'protective' cholesterol and lower LDL 'harmful' cholesterol.

The Mediterranean diet is particularly high in omega-3 fats, which are a type of polyunsaturated fat found in marine foods and plants. Omega-3 fats may help reduce blood clotting, interrupt the build-up of plaque and inflammation in the arteries, lower heart rate, lower triglycerides and reduce blood pressure. Omega-3 fats are found in oily fish including tuna, salmon and sardines with smaller amounts in other white fish such as barramundi and flathead and seafood like scallops and mussels. Plant sources of omega-3 fats include nuts (walnuts) and seeds (flaxseeds and chia).

Research shows that replacing saturated fats with monounsaturated and omega-3 fats contributes to a reduction in heart disease and stroke risk. The Mediterranean diet's emphasis on monounsaturated fats means that it has a high monounsaturated-to-saturated fat ratio.

SATURATED AND TRANS FATS

Saturated and trans fats contribute to heart disease by increasing total blood cholesterol and LDL cholesterol. Saturated fat comes from animal-based foods such as meat, butter and cream, as well as coconut-based foods. Trans fats are formed by the partial hydrogenation of vegetable oils to produce margarine and vegetable shortenings, and these are found in processed foods such as biscuits, cakes and chips. Saturated and trans fats increase LDL cholesterol and reduce HDL cholesterol. The Mediterranean diet includes only small amounts of lean meats; the more common proteins include fish, lean poultry and beans and legumes, and includes very little processed food.

DIETARY CHOLESTEROL

The cholesterol in food, or 'dietary cholesterol', only has a small effect on the level of cholesterol in the blood. Cholesterol-rich foods, including offal (liver, kidneys and brains) and eggs, can be eaten as part of a balanced Mediterranean diet. The Heart Foundation of Australia suggests that people who have type 2 diabetes or high blood cholesterol should limit eggs to seven per week.

Risk factor 3: Blood pressure

Blood pressure is the pressure of your blood against the walls of your arteries, and it goes up and down depending on what you are doing. A measure of 120/80mmHg is ideal. Blood pressure consistently above the normal range (greater than 140/90 mmHg) is referred to as high blood pressure, and that is a strong risk factor for heart disease.

The impact of diet and its components on blood pressure have been investigated since the 1940s, when scientists became interested in the association between sodium intake and elevated blood pressure. Since then, several dietary approaches to protect against elevated blood pressure have emerged, such as lowering salt and alcohol intake and increasing plant food intakes.

Since the 1990s, elevated blood pressure has been acknowledged as a major contributor to the global burden of disease, and today it remains one of the five largest contributors. Lowering blood pressure levels is associated with reduced risk of many chronic conditions, including heart disease and cardiovascular mortality. Importantly, life-course studies have shown that early-life eating habits beginning in infancy impact on blood pressure by early school-age, suggesting that early intervention is needed in order to stem the tide of elevated blood pressure globally. More recently, a growing body of evidence shows that particular dietary patterns, including traditional diets, and not just dietary components, influence blood pressure. These are increasingly promoted as 'heart-healthy diets' and are reflected in the national dietary guidelines of many countries. The most researched of the blood pressure-lowering diets are the DASH and Mediterranean diets.

While the Dietary Approaches to Stop Hypertension (aka DASH Diet), is similar to a Mediterranean diet, it also focuses on lowering salt. The DASH diet was developed to lower blood pressure, but the advantage of the Mediterranean diet is that it has proven to be sustainable and palatable over thousands of years. It can also be easily adapted to suit non-Mediterranean populations using the principles outlined on pages 10–11. As illustrated in this section, this diet has demonstrated benefits well beyond its beneficial effects on blood pressure.

A recent review summarising the effects of a Mediterranean diet on blood pressure concluded this dietary pattern has a favourable effect on blood pressure. Among recent studies, adherence to a Mediterranean diet was also associated with lower blood pressure in 12-year-olds. In several studies on high-risk individuals, most with treated hypertension, a Mediterranean diet supplemented with extra-virgin olive oil or nuts reduced blood pressure. In an Australian study, adults who consumed a Mediterranean diet for 6 months had a reduction in systolic blood pressure. Although the size of the blood pressure-lowering effect of the Mediterranean diet is yet to be quantified in different populations, based on current evidence the effect will be favourable.

If you are concerned about your weight or any of the other risk factors, you should consult your doctor or an accredited practising dietitian.

Risk factor 4: Obesity

Obesity – defined as having excessive amounts of body fat in relation to height – is associated with an increased risk of many chronic diseases, including type 2 diabetes and heart disease. Abdominal fat in particular is well recognised as a major risk factor for type 2 diabetes and heart disease. The visceral fat that accumulates around the viscera or internal abdominal organs is more harmful than subcutaneous fat under the skin or around the hips and thighs because visceral fat cells are metabolically active. They produce inflammatory chemicals called cytokines and adipokines which have pro-atherosclerotic properties and anti-insulin action.

We also know that accumulation of fat around our body organs promotes tissue inflammation. This sustained inflammation has also been shown to play a key role in the initiation, progression and destabilisation of atherosclerotic plaques.

Waist circumference is commonly used to assess whether someone has excessive abdominal fat: a waist circumference above 102 cm for men and 88 cm for women is considered excessive and increases their risk of chronic disease. Weight loss through diet and exercise is the only way to tackle this. In clinical studies, the Mediterranean diet has consistently been shown to be effective for long-term, sustainable weight loss as it is highly palatable and satisfying. The PREDIMED study found that those following a Mediterranean diet had a greater reduction in weight, lower waist circumference, lower blood pressure and lower levels of inflammation compared with those following a low-fat diet.

Risk factor 5: Type 2 diabetes

Diabetes is a serious condition and one of the fastest-growing diseases across the world. There are three types: type 1, type 2 and gestational diabetes, with type 2 diabetes being the most common – around 90 per cent of people with diabetes have this form. Type 2 diabetes is strongly associated with poor diet and lifestyle, though genetic predisposition also plays a role. Though there is no cure for diabetes, the condition can be well controlled with a healthy diet and regular physical activity. In some cases, diabetes medication may be required.

In a healthy state, blood sugar levels rise after a meal and the pancreas releases the hormone insulin that helps shift the glucose into cells to be used for energy. The liver can also produce glucose. With diabetes, however, your body cannot control glucose levels as the pancreas does not produce sufficient insulin or there is 'insulin resistance', which means the insulin is not working effectively. This leads to chronic hyperglycaemia and complications.

Over 80 per cent of people with diabetes are overweight or obese, and a modest weight loss of 5–10 per cent of their body weight can significantly improve control of diabetes and reduce their risk of heart disease. The Mediterranean diet has consistently proven to be effective in the prevention and management of type 2 diabetes. The PREDIMED study found that people following a Mediterranean diet were about 50 per cent less likely to develop type 2 diabetes compared with those on a low-fat diet.

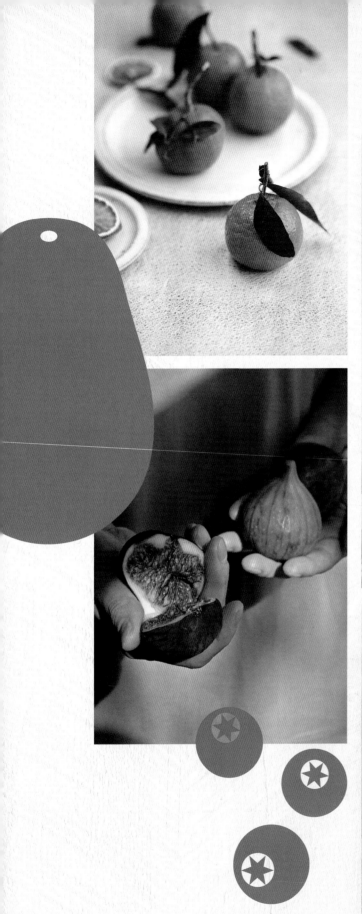
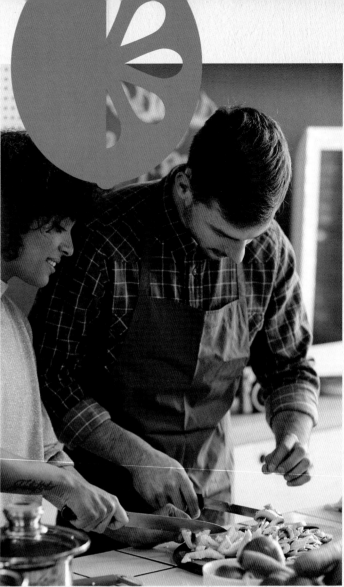
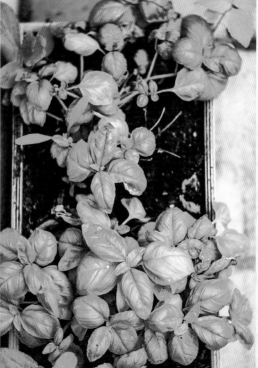

PART 2

Following
a Mediterranean diet

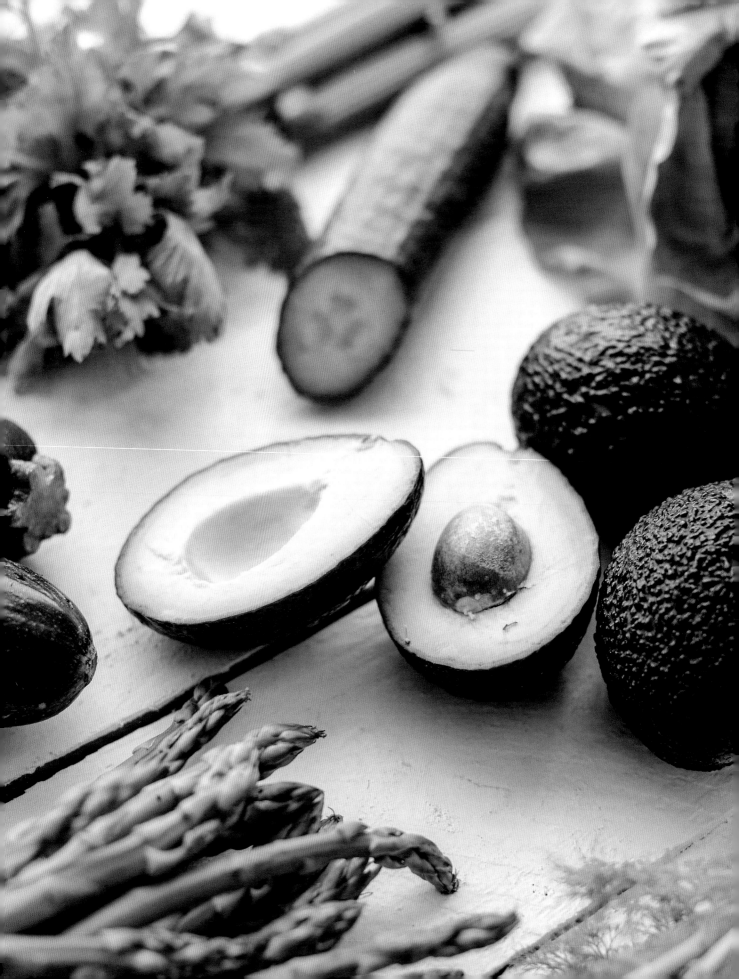

Heart healthy, tasty *and* satisfying

'Your brain is a pig: How evolution has primed us to gorge ourselves on fattening foods'. This is the title of an article published on Canadian news site CBC.ca. It was written by Professor Gordon Orians, a professor emeritus of evolutionary biology at the University of Washington in Seattle. The pig statement may be alarming, but it really does help to explain why following a healthy eating pattern can be so difficult to sustain. It also explains how, despite good intentions, our brains will often guide us to make food choices that are high in energy (kilojoules), fat and sugar.

As humans, we evolved under conditions of food scarcity where our principle occupation was finding and consuming enough energy to stay alive. We are genetically engineered to prefer or seek out high-fat foods because fats are more energy dense – fat contains three times more energy per gram compared to carbohydrate-rich foods.

Not only was food scarce, but it also required a lot of energy (exercise/effort) to obtain and prepare. A few indigenous populations such as Aboriginal Australians, indigenous Eskimo populations in Alaska and, today, tribes in Ooty, India, still live a traditional hunter-gatherer lifestyle. When they are in their natural environments, they do not experience heart disease and diabetes. However, when they migrate to cities and change their dietary habits to consume processed foods and become less active, they rapidly develop diabetes and heart disease and at a faster rate than the populations already living in these cities.

A Mediterranean diet is not quite a hunter-gatherer way of eating, but it does have many of the qualities that would be experienced by traditional hunter-gatherers: home gardens, plenty of vegetables and leafy greens, nuts, dried fruits, game meats and foods that are much less processed and therefore take lots of effort to produce.

The beauty of the Mediterranean diet is, relative to the Western diet, when we eat this way, it keeps us fuller for longer. And this is attributed to the bulkiness of the diet, which contains a high quantity of plant foods, especially leafy vegetables that have a high-water content. Foods with a high-water content are bulky and have fewer kilojoules per 100 g than foods with low-water content. In addition, foods that are carbohydrate-rich have lower kilojoules, as carbohydrates have a 16 kj/gram energy content versus fats, which have a 37 kj/gram energy content.

Legumes, which are full of fibre, also have a lower calorie/kilojoule value per meal compared to a meal rich in animal proteins and fats. A dietary pattern that has lower energy density has less energy (or kilojoules) per gram of food eaten. There is a vast difference in energy density between a bulky Mediterranean meal compared to a highly processed meal.

Which meal is more filling?

Here are two examples of typical lunches,
each provides around 2400kj (600 calories).

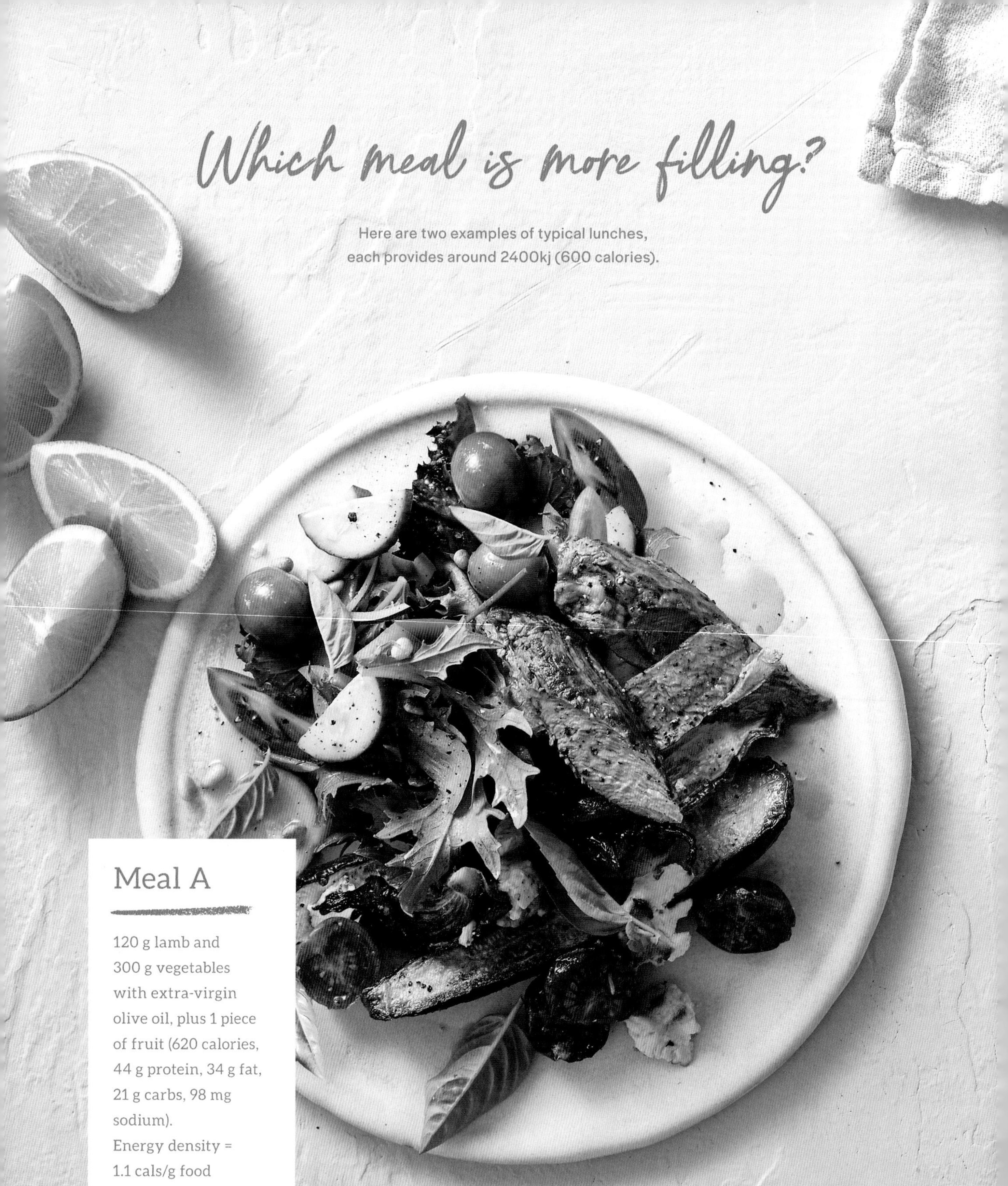

Meal A

120 g lamb and
300 g vegetables
with extra-virgin
olive oil, plus 1 piece
of fruit (620 calories,
44 g protein, 34 g fat,
21 g carbs, 98 mg
sodium).
Energy density =
1.1 cals/g food

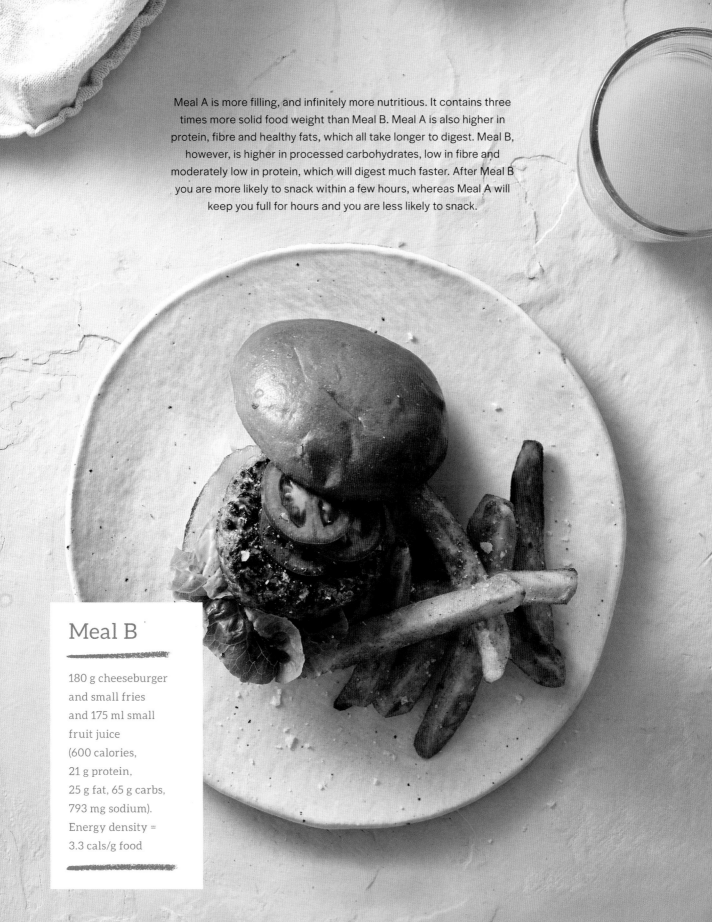

Meal A is more filling, and infinitely more nutritious. It contains three times more solid food weight than Meal B. Meal A is also higher in protein, fibre and healthy fats, which all take longer to digest. Meal B, however, is higher in processed carbohydrates, low in fibre and moderately low in protein, which will digest much faster. After Meal B you are more likely to snack within a few hours, whereas Meal A will keep you full for hours and you are less likely to snack.

Meal B

180 g cheeseburger
and small fries
and 175 ml small
fruit juice
(600 calories,
21 g protein,
25 g fat, 65 g carbs,
793 mg sodium).
Energy density =
3.3 cals/g food

Translating the Mediterranean diet for everyone

The beauty of the Mediterranean diet is that you don't have to live in the Mediterranean to enjoy eating this way – with a few ingredient swaps and tweaks, the principles and core philosophies of this diet can be applied to make it suitable for many countries, cultures and ethnicities.

To ensure that the benefits can be enjoyed by Australians and other populations, it is important to be flexible so as many people as possible can follow and enjoy the Mediterranean diet, which includes good food and health.

The Mediterranean diet is not just a diet, it's also a way of life, with many social and cultural components. The philosophy of eating together and sharing meals is at the core of the Mediterranean diet, and there is great emphasis placed on family meals. There is also a difference in cooking methods and use of ingredients, with traditional cooking practices (e.g. slow-cooking), seasonal foods and use of herbs and spices all being important components of this way of eating.

Many foods consumed as part of a traditional Mediterranean diet – such as wild leafy plants like sow thistle and dandelion, snails or wild hare – may not be readily available in Australia or suitable for certain people depending on their culture or religion. Consequently, different foods need to be swapped in order to maintain alliance and nutritional profile with the principles of the Mediterranean diet.

When looking at tweaking the diet for your particular region, culture, likes and dislikes, there are four areas to consider:

1
Eating patterns:
Understand the health benefits of each of the 10 key principles of the Mediterranean diet (pages 10–11); understand why each ingredient is important, and what its benefits are.

2
Food availability:
What is locally grown and available where you are?

3
Acceptability:
What food options suit your culture, ethnicity and food preferences?

4
Cuisine:
How can you prepare these ingredients in a way that ties in with your culture and cooking style, and also preserve the benefits of the way these ingredients are prepared, combined and cooked?

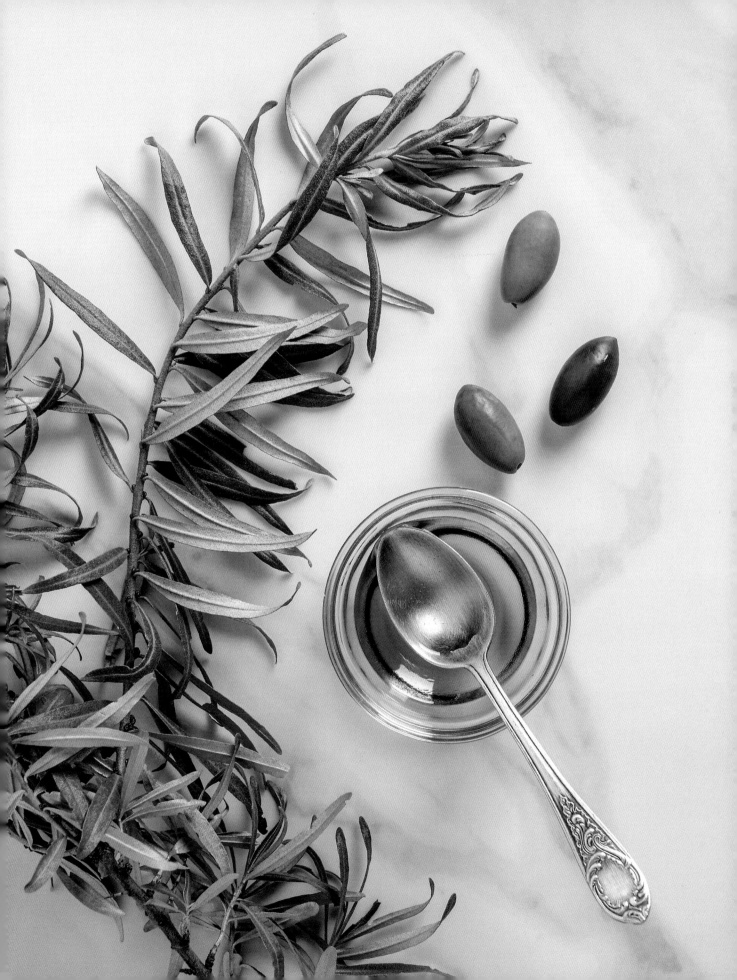

The Australian dietary guidelines and the Mediterranean diet

In Australia, when my colleagues and I translate a traditional Mediterranean diet for our Australian patients, it is also important for us to consider how our recommendations may differ from the Australian dietary guidelines (ADG).

The ADGs recommend that foods from the following five groups are consumed:

1 Vegetables, including different types and colours, and legumes/beans

2 Fruits

3 Grain (cereal) foods, mostly wholegrain and/or high cereal-fibre varieties, such as breads, cereals, rice, pasta, noodles, polenta, couscous, oats, quinoa and barley

4 Lean meats and poultry, fish, eggs, tofu, nuts and seeds, and legumes/beans

5 Milk, yoghurt, cheese and/or their alternatives, mostly reduced-fat (note that reduced-fat milks are not suitable for children under the age of two)

Here's how the two diets compare. →

How the ADGs compare to the Mediterranean diet

ADG Guideline Number	ADG recommendations	Mediterranean diet
Guideline 1	To achieve and maintain a healthy weight, you must be physically active and choose amounts of nutritious food and drinks to meet your energy needs.	Consistent with the ADG's recommendations (see the Functional Pyramid on page 62).
Guideline 2	Enjoy a wide variety of nutritious foods from the five groups every day and drink plenty of water.	Mostly consistent with the ADGs, with these key differences: • Extra-virgin olive oil is the main added fat in cooked dishes and salads. • Minimal consumption of red meat. • Moderate consumption of poultry, eggs and pork. • Full-fat dairy (especially fermented dairy such as yoghurt and feta) eaten moderately. • Alcohol in the form of wine, consumed in moderation.
Guideline 3	Limit intake of foods containing saturated fat, added salt, added sugars and alcohol. Limit intake of foods high in saturated fat such as many biscuits, cakes, pastries, pies, processed meats, commercial burgers, pizza, fried foods, potato chips, crisps and other savoury snacks. a. Replace high-fat foods which contain predominantly saturated fats such as butter, cream, cooking margarine, coconut and palm oil with foods that contain predominantly polyunsaturated and monounsaturated fats, such as oils, spreads, nut butters/pastes and avocado. Low-fat diets are not suitable for children under the age of two. b. Limit intake of foods and drinks containing added salt. Read labels to choose lower-sodium options among similar foods. Do not add salt to foods in cooking or at the table. c. Limit intake of foods and drinks containing added sugars such as confectionary, sugar-sweetened soft drinks and cordials, fruit drinks, vitamin waters, energy and sports drinks. d. If you choose to drink alcohol, limit intake. For women who are pregnant, planning a pregnancy or breastfeeding, not drinking alcohol is the safest option.	Mostly consistent with the ADGs: The Mediterranean diet principles include a focus on fresh cooked foods, snacks are usually fresh and dried fruit, nuts and yoghurt, and sweets for special occasions only. a. Key differences to the ADGs is that the Mediterranean diet uses extra-virgin olive oil as the main added fat. Other fats and oils used (e.g. margarines, seed oils) are not usually used. The Mediterranean diet is a healthy high-fat diet. b. Consistent: The Mediterranean diet is naturally lower in salt (except for olives, pickles and cheeses) as foods are cooked fresh and there is little salt from processed foods. c. Consistent with the ADGs, sweets are for special occasions only. d. Different to ADGs. A traditional Mediterranean diet includes wine (preferably red) with meals, in moderation, and usually 1–2 glasses per day. Recommendations for pregnant or breastfeeding women are the same as the ADGs.
Guideline 4	Encourage, support and promote breastfeeding.	Breastfeeding is the mainstay for feeding infants.
Guideline 5	Care for your food; prepare and store it safely.	Consistent: The Mediterranean people have used traditional methods of preparing, cooking and storing food to minimise spoilage such as drying, pickling and using olive oil to layer over foods (e.g. olives, tomato paste) to prevent moulds growing.

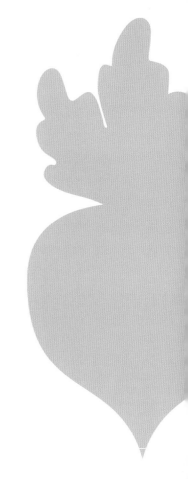

THE HEART FOUNDATION'S GUIDELINES

The Heart Foundation is a national leading authority in research into the prevention and treatment of heart disease in Australia. It is an authoritative charitable non-government organisation that publishes guidelines for the management of heart disease for doctors, dietitians and other health professionals. The Heart Foundation recently commissioned an extensive review that examined a number of different diets and their link to improved health outcomes for people with heart disease. Rather than focusing on individual nutrients such as fats, salt and sugar, this current approach to guidelines focuses on healthy patterns of eating. The Mediterranean diet is called out as a key diet that is protective for heart disease. Another healthy diet this review highlighted is the DASH diet.

The new Heart Foundation diet guidelines for the management of heart disease are very similar to the Mediterranean diet. The guidelines include consuming plenty of vegetables, fruits and wholegrains, eating a variety of healthy protein foods such as fish and legumes and smaller serves of poultry, consuming healthy fats from nuts, seeds, olives and their oils, and using herbs and spices to flavour foods instead of salt.

Where the Heart Foundation guidelines differ to the Mediterranean diet is in its recommendation to eat lean red meat 1–3 times per week (350 g maximum per week), and use a variety of oils from nuts, seeds or olives.

In contrast, the Mediterranean diet includes less red meat and focuses on extra-virgin olive oil as the primary added fat.

For people at high risk of heart disease — those that have already experienced a heart attack, have type 2 diabetes or have a high cholesterol level — the Heart Foundation guidelines also recommend low-fat dairy foods and limiting eggs to seven per week.

Supporting your microbiome

As we discussed in Part 1, maintaining a healthy gut is integral to lowering inflammation in the body and maintaining good health. And the many prebiotic foods in the Mediterranean diet are rich in different types of fibre, FODMAPS (fermentable oligosaccharides, polysaccharides and polyols), resistant starch (page 40), polyphenols (plant-based antioxidants), plant proteins and unsaturated fats, all of which act like fertiliser promoting the growth of beneficial bacteria that ferment these foods in the gut to produce beneficial metabolites such as short-chain fatty acids (propionate, butyrate, acetate).

Metabolites produced by beneficial bacteria are important because they help to heal the gut, which in turn stops any inflammatory toxins from entering the blood and causing low-grade systemic inflammation. Metabolites can also have a beneficial effect on our metabolism and physiology – they help to reduce blood glucose, cholesterol and appetite. In contrast, animal foods high in saturated fat, branched chain amino acids, carnitine and choline undergo bacterial putrefaction in the gut resulting in toxic metabolites that can damage the gut and contribute to low-grade systemic inflammation. They are also potential carcinogens and toxins to the heart and blood vessels.

Animal studies have shown that consumption of emulsifiers, found in processed foods, can have a negative effect on health by altering the microbiome (thus reducing the friendly bacteria and increasing the toxic bacteria) and increasing blood sugars and causing overeating and weight gain. There are very few studies in humans, but early studies show that eating highly processed foods can lead to overeating and higher levels of cholesterol and inflammatory markers.

PREBIOTIC- AND PROBIOTIC-RICH FOODS

A key benefit of the Mediterranean diet in maintaining a healthy microbiome is the abundance of foods with probiotic and prebiotic functions. Probiotics (meaning 'for life' in Greek) are living microorganisms that provide health benefits when consumed. Your body is full of bacteria, both good and bad, and this community of bacteria is called the microbiome.

Prebiotics

Prebiotics are dietary fibres that help feed the friendly bacteria in the gut. These fibres are found in a number of foods and are usually resistant to digestion. Because of this, they are able to reach the lower gut (large bowel) undigested. They are consumed by the friendly bacteria (probiotics) via fermentation.

Probiotics

Probiotics are live bacteria, similar to those already found in the microbiome colony in the gut, but they can also be yeasts. Common probiotic bacteria groups include Lactobacillus and Bifidobacterium. They are available as supplements (in various forms) and are produced from foods by bacterial fermentation. Any food that has been fermented is likely to contain probiotics. Probiotics are often called 'good' or 'helpful' bacteria because they help to keep your gut healthy.

Key prebiotics and probiotics ingredients in the Mediterranean diet

Prebiotics

Dark green leafy veggies, especially dandelion leaves

Cabbage, beetroot, carrots

Artichoke, asparagus, green beans

Garlic, onions, leeks, spring onions

Tomatoes, eggplant, zucchini, pumpkin, sweet potato

Fennel bulbs

Peas and split peas

Lentils, chickpeas, beans, lupins

Barley, spelt, wheat bread (toasted), oats (raw), gnocchi, couscous

Potato, rice, pasta (cooked and cooled*)

Apples, pears, plums, berries, figs

Nectarines, apricots, white peaches, watermelons, pomegranates

Lemon, oranges, grapefruit

Pistachios, hazelnuts, almonds, walnuts, tahini

Olives and extra-virgin olive oil

Herbs and spices

Grapes, grape vinegar, red wine, spirits made from grapes (raki)

Probiotics

Olives

Feta and goat's cheese

Kefalograviera (similar to gruyere)

Kefalotiri

Mizithra (whey cheese)

Gouda and cheddar

Greek-style yoghurt

Trahana** (fermented wheat in sour milk)

Sourdough bread

When cooked and then cooled, the starch in potato, rice or pasta forms resistant starch. This type of starch is not digested in the small bowel and travels to the large bowel, where it can be consumed by friendly bacteria.

**This is a common traditional breakfast dish or light dinner eaten with bread and feta.*

The Dietary Inflammatory Index

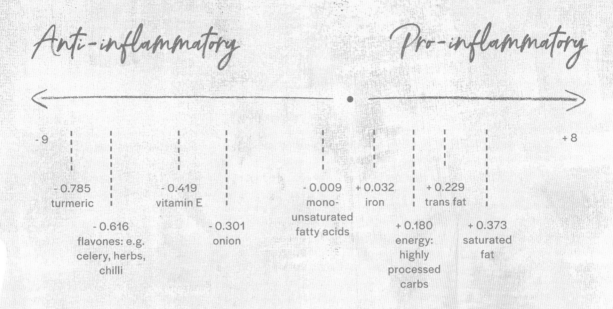

Anti-inflammatory

Pro-inflammatory

-9

+8

- 0.785
turmeric

- 0.616
flavones: e.g.
celery, herbs,
chilli

- 0.419
vitamin E

- 0.301
onion

- 0.009
mono-
unsaturated
fatty acids

+ 0.032
iron

+ 0.180
energy:
highly
processed
carbs

+ 0.229
trans fat

+ 0.373
saturated
fat

THE DIETARY INFLAMMATORY INDEX

The Dietary Inflammatory Index (DII) is a new and novel way of measuring the health properties of diets. It incorporates 45 different foods and ingredients that have pro-inflammatory and anti-inflammatory properties. And our studies have shown that the traditional Cretan Mediterranean diet scores the highest in terms of anti-inflammatory potential, much better than the well-known low-fat diet.

The above diagram shows how the score works with foods containing animal (saturated) fats and cholesterol, and highly processed foods (which include trans fats, and highly processed carbohydrates) scoring high on the pro-inflammatory scale.

On the other hand, foods that are typical of a Mediterranean diet such as extra-virgin olive oil (rich in monounsaturated fat and polyphenols), leafy vegetables, tomatoes, onions, garlic, legumes, herbs and spices such as ginger, turmeric, saffron, score high on the anti-inflammatory scale.

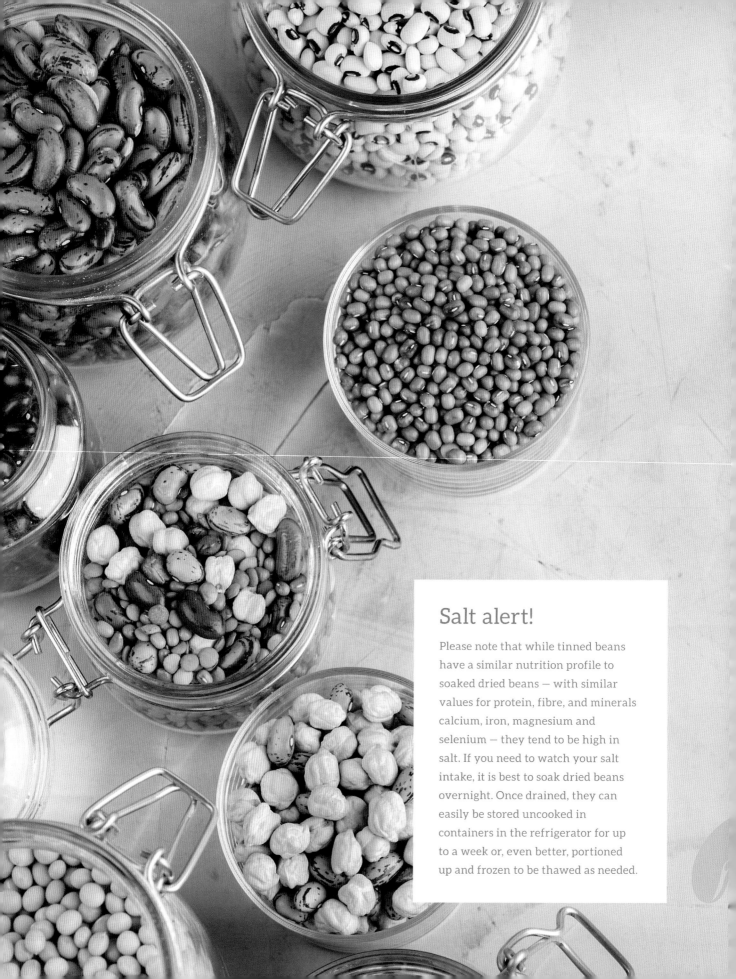

Salt alert!

Please note that while tinned beans have a similar nutrition profile to soaked dried beans — with similar values for protein, fibre, and minerals calcium, iron, magnesium and selenium — they tend to be high in salt. If you need to watch your salt intake, it is best to soak dried beans overnight. Once drained, they can easily be stored uncooked in containers in the refrigerator for up to a week or, even better, portioned up and frozen to be thawed as needed.

Make legumes the hero of the dish

If you're transitioning to a Mediterranean diet from a typical Western diet, one of the biggest changes for you will likely be getting used to eating more beans and legumes. Though legumes such as lentils, chickpeas and beans form a staple part of many diets around the world, they only make occasional appearances in the typical Western diet.

Legumes are an important source of protein in vegetarian diets and people from the Mediterranean, especially Greeks who follow a Greek orthodox religion, will often consume a vegan diet for up to 150 days of the year. This form of religious fasting also acts in a way to detoxify the body from high-fat animal foods and therefore may have additional health benefits. During those vegan fasting periods, there is a strong reliance on legumes as the main source of protein.

Learning how to prepare and cook legumes will be very important in order for you to make the Mediterranean diet part of your life in the long term. An easy way to start doing this is by adding a few tablespoons of drained, tinned chickpeas or lentils to salads and stews. Many of the recipes in this book include legumes, and you'll find beans added to stews to bulk them out, boost fibre content and keep the portions of meat small — think of them as 'meat extenders'.

Try to incorporate legumes at least twice a week and go meat-free for two days a week (see the meal plan on page 68 for a 'Meatless Monday' idea). Keeping a variety of tinned legumes in the pantry such as chickpeas, cannellini beans, butter beans and four-bean mix will make them easy to include in all kinds of meals.

If you find incorporating legumes hard, another easy way to start introducing them into your diet is with lupin flour. Lupin is a special legume. It is the world's richest natural source of combined plant protein and fibre. It is more nutritious than other legumes with double the amount of protein and fibre and negligible anti-nutritional factors like lectins and phytates, which can reduce absorption of nutrients.

Lupin is traditionally consumed as a boiled bean snack in brine in Greece, especially in Crete. It can also be purchased in this form in Australia in some specialty shops.

In some parts of Greece, lupin is milled into a fine flour and combined with wheat flour to make bread, biscuits, pancakes and pies.

Replacing about half the wheat flour in recipes with lupin flour will dramatically improve the protein and fibre content (for recipe ideas check out profkourisnutrition.com.au). Also, lupin flour does not need cooking, so it can be added to smoothies and yoghurt. It can also be added to stews to thicken them or used as a binding agent. Lupin, however, is an allergen and it cross-reacts with peanuts. People with nut and soy allergies should avoid lupin.

When embarking on a Mediterranean diet, it's worth remembering that because of its high plant food content, especially legumes, you are likely to experience more flatulence than normal and possibly softer stools until your gut microbiome adapts to the change.

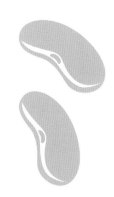

Extra-virgin olive oil: a Mediterranean hero

Olive oil is ubiquitous across the Mediterranean and forms the basis of a healthy Mediterranean diet. Because this ingredient is such a crucial component of this diet and lifestyle, it's important to know the difference between a high-quality oil and a low-quality oil in order to ensure you are getting all the health benefits this natural ingredient can provide.

In July 2011, Standards Australia introduced The Australian Standard for Olive Oils and Olive Pomace Oils (AS-5264-2011) to differentiate between high-quality extra-virgin olive oil and lower-class oils with little or no health benefits.

To better understand the different grades of olive oil it is important to first understand how olive oil is processed.

Natural olive oil is the fruit juice of olives, and it is extracted through mechanical separation (crushing and mixing) at a low temperature (less than 30°C) and filtered. No chemical extraction is used for natural olive oils. The oil is then tested for flavour and acidity. The grades of olive oil, from highest to lowest, are as follows.

GRADES OF OLIVE OIL

Extra-virgin olive oil (also called 'cold pressed' or 'first pressed'): this oil is free of trans fats, has no flavour defects, is highest in polyphenols/antioxidants and has a free fatty acid content of <0.8% (low acidity).

Virgin olive oil: this oil is a lower grade and has some minor flavour defects, lower polyphenols/antioxidants and a free fatty acid content of 0.8–2% (moderate acidity).

Lampanate oil: this is not fit for human consumption. It has too many defects, free fatty acid content greater than 2% (high acidity) and is usually spoiled due to damaged fruit or a delay in processing. This oil is used in chemically refined oils.

REFINED OILS AND BLENDED OILS

Refined oil: chemically refined, clear in colour with no polyphenols.

Olive oil: often called '100% pure olive oil', 'light oil' or 'extra-light oil'. It is a combination of refined olive oil with 5–15% virgin olive oil added to it. The lighter or paler oils have less virgin olive oil. This oil is very low in polyphenols/antioxidants and has a bland flavour.

Pomace oil: produced from the waste product (pomace) that is removed at the first phase of olive oil pressing. This oil includes the crushed pips, flesh and skin of the olive and damaged fruit. The oil is extracted using solvents. This oil is not for human consumption and is used for technical purposes only.

CAN YOU COOK WITH EXTRA-VIRGIN OLIVE OIL?

In short, yes! There is a common misconception that extra-virgin olive oil should only be consumed raw, and that when it is cooked the health properties disappear. This is not true. In fact, if you were to ask an elderly Mediterranean person, they would argue that there has only ever been one olive oil in their kitchen for dressing salads, cooking casseroles, baking dishes in the oven, frying and even making sweets, and that is extra-virgin olive oil.

It is believed that fats and oils that have a low smoke point (the temperature at which the oil produces a thin continuous stream of bluish smoke) are not ideal for high-temperature cooking such as frying (temperatures greater than 180°C). Extra-virgin olive oil generally has a lower smoke point than other oils such as seed oils, coconut oil and rice bran oil, so it is often not used for frying as people believe it is not safe.

To prove whether extra-virgin olive oil was safe to cook with, a team of researchers in Australia tested nine common oils found in the supermarket, including Australian extra-virgin olive oil, olive oil (refined blend), canola oil, rice bran oil, grapeseed oil, coconut oil, peanut oil, sunflower oil and avocado oil. They heated these oils up to 240°C and then heated them for 6 hours at 180°C to show the effects higher than normal temperatures and longer cooking periods would have on the production of harmful chemicals in the oils. The study measured smoke point and the production of trans fats and polar compounds caused by oxidation of the oils – these are the harmful changes that occur with heating.

The study showed that extra-virgin olive oil performed better than the other common cooking oils. It produced less trans fats, retained higher levels of antioxidants and, most importantly, had lower levels of the potentially harmful polar compounds that have a detrimental effect on human health.

The extra-virgin olive oil was protected from oxidation due to the stable fatty acid profile (mainly monounsaturated fats and low in polyunsaturated fats) and high content of polyphenols with antioxidant properties.

Use your extra-virgin olive oil liberally for all cooking purposes!

A sustainable way of eating for the planet and your wallet

As we touched on in Part 1, not only is the Mediterranean diet healthier and more satisfying from a nutritional point of view, it's also more satisfying from an environmental point of view because it's more environmentally sustainable than the Western diet. When you look at the tips commonly given to people who want to eat more sustainability, you can see the many ways the Mediterranean diet ties in a more sustainable approach to food shopping and eating.

Eat more sustainably by

- Consuming more plants including vegetables, legumes and nuts.

- Eating less meat – replace it with fish and legumes.

- Including more wholefoods in each meal, and fewer processed foods.

- Eating a variety of foods and buying locally produced, seasonal foods.

- Wasting less food by buying only what you need.

- Buying food with less packaging.

A common misconception is that a healthy diet is more expensive than an unhealthy diet. This can certainly be true if you consider a healthy diet to consist of premium cuts of meat, wild-caught fish, premium imported ingredients bought from boutique groceries and handpicked organic vegetables.

However, a plant-based diet with sustainably sourced ingredients from local producers that are minimally processed with less packaging can also be economical.

An analysis of average weekly food costs in a study our team completed in people with mild depression called the SMILES Study showed that those following a Mediterranean-style diet were spending $112 per week on food compared with people following their usual diet spending $138 per week – a $26 difference /week). Remarkably, the people following the Mediterranean-style eating pattern had significantly lower depression scores at the end of the study and almost one-third went into remission. The study was aimed at improving the health profile of people with depression as there is growing evidence that people with depression have increased risk of heart disease and other chronic poor-lifestyle related diseases.

The Mediterranean eating pattern included healthy snacks in between meals such as fresh fruit and nuts instead of highly processed high-sugar high-fat snacks and drinks. There were also more fresh-cooked, home-prepared meals in the Mediterranean pattern instead of highly processed take-away foods.

The following habits for shopping and cooking will help you achieve a Mediterranean diet on a budget:

Buy vegetables in bulk and aim to consume them within a week so they don't spoil.

Use up the fresh leafy vegetables first by preparing salads and also making soups that can be frozen.

Buy fruits and vegetables in season as they are often more abundant and on sale. These days our fresh food supply is fairly continuous as foods are transported from all over the world, so we don't often notice the seasonality of fruits and vegetables; however, price is a determinant as imported fresh fruits and vegetables are much more expensive and have a high carbon footprint.

Don't overlook the ugly vegetables. They may be imperfect to look at, but they have the same nutritional value and are often a lot cheaper than their perfectly proportioned counterparts.

Try to make a habit of making your own stock with your leftover vegetables so that you have it on hand when you need it. This will save you money and help you cut back on salt.

Buy dried beans in bulk from markets or grocers, or even in bags from the supermarket. Get into the habit of soaking them overnight and then draining them before dividing them into 250 g (wet weight) portions to cook later. Beans that are soaked can easily be frozen and then used up as needed. This will save money and is also an excellent way to cut down on salt, as tinned beans are quite salty.

Use legumes (beans) as meat-extenders in casseroles and stews (see recipes on pages 195, 202 and 215). Doing this means you can cut down on the meat serve per person and add beans to extend the meal adding protein from legumes. This also boosts the fibre and makes the meal more filling.

Choose cheaper cuts of meat for use in casseroles and stews. The meat just needs cooking a little longer before you add the vegetables or beans to the dish (see Beef cassoulet on page 215).

Choose small fin fish such as fresh sardines, pilchards or other small fish. Best to buy at the markets. These fish are not only cheaper than larger fish, but they are also higher in omega-3 fats.

Buy olive oil in bulk such as in 3- or 4-litre tins and store in a cool dry place. Decant into small, dark glass bottles for using. Check the price per 100 ml and you will see it is always cheaper to buy it this way, even when it's not on sale.

Buy dried herbs in bulk rather than in small bottles or packets. Herbs are used abundantly in Mediterranean dishes so you will need larger quantities. Bags of 50 g in the supermarkets are much cheaper, but if you are adventurous, visit a Mediterranean (or Middle Eastern) wholesaler and buy larger quantities. You will also find greater varieties of herbs and spices at these types of shop.

Tomato purée is another staple, and **using fresh, grated tomatoes**, especially when they are cheaper and in season is best as the flavour they impart is much fresher and less acidic, and there is no added salt in fresh tomatoes. Tinned tomatoes and bottled puréed tomatoes are great to have in the pantry as a back-up.

Buy nuts in 1 kg bags, or in bulk from grocers or markets. This is much cheaper than buying small 30 g pre-packs, and an added bonus is that this cuts down on packaging.

Home-grown heart health

We can learn many lessons from long-living cultures. The healthy immigrant effect (HIE), whereby migrants are healthier compared to the host population is widely documented and has been observed among migrant groups globally. However, over time, after increasing years of living in their new country, most migrant groups tend to adopt the diet and lifestyle factors of their host population. Over time, migrants also tend to develop the same disease patterns of the host country, and this is often due to picking up the diet and lifestyle habits of their new home.

Interestingly, our research has found that migrants from Greece have resisted changing their habits even after spending years in Australia. Instead, they have retained many of their traditional Mediterranean diet habits. We understand that this resistance to change has led to fewer deaths from heart disease and healthy longevity in this migrant group.

In a study led by Dr Antonia Thodis, our Mediterranean diet research group from La Trobe University along with Harokopio University in Athens, Greece, examined the health characteristics of Greek migrants who have spent more than 40 years in Australia. We found that 80 per cent of these migrants were 'home-grown food gardeners', i.e. they maintain a backyard garden to cultivate fruit and/or vegetables. The typical fruits and vegetables grown by the Greek migrants in our study included citrus fruits (especially lemons), tomatoes, onions, garlic and leafy green vegetables (especially bitter leafy greens). Other produce commonly grown by our study subjects included cabbages, cauliflower and broccoli and apples, pears and stone fruit.

Growing their own fruits and vegetables had a huge impact on their diet as their home garden provided over half the fruit and vegetable supply for the household. When we examined their physical activity patterns, we found that gardening was the most common daily activity, especially among the elderly Greek men. Maintaining a fruit and vegetable garden requires a higher level of physical activity than keeping a flower garden, and this may be another important healthy habit that has assisted the health status of Greek migrants.

Gardening has two key benefits: it gets people moving around and exposes them to sunlight, thus increasing vitamin D production in the skin, both of which are protective for heart disease and other chronic diseases. As well as increasing physical activity and improving vitamin D status, growing your own fruit and vegetables improves the quality of your diet and saves money!

Few studies have investigated the role of backyard fruit and vegetable gardens among migrants to Australia, yet this practice has sociocultural significance in terms of maintaining links with their homeland and could be viewed as a marker of resilience to acculturation.

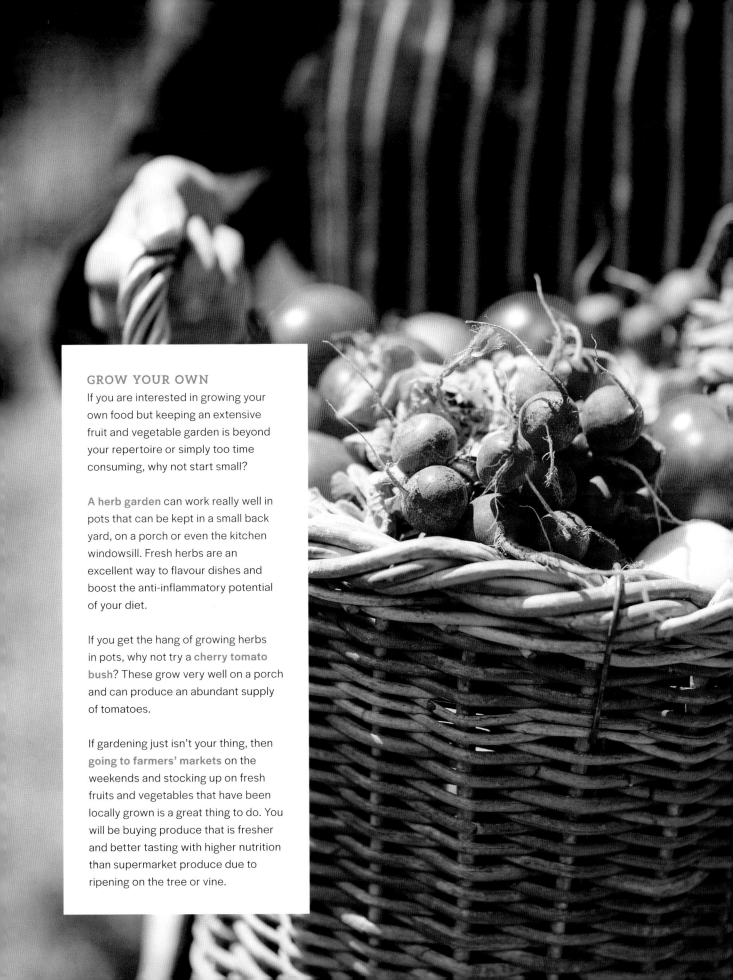

GROW YOUR OWN

If you are interested in growing your own food but keeping an extensive fruit and vegetable garden is beyond your repertoire or simply too time consuming, why not start small?

A herb garden can work really well in pots that can be kept in a small back yard, on a porch or even the kitchen windowsill. Fresh herbs are an excellent way to flavour dishes and boost the anti-inflammatory potential of your diet.

If you get the hang of growing herbs in pots, why not try a **cherry tomato bush**? These grow very well on a porch and can produce an abundant supply of tomatoes.

If gardening just isn't your thing, then **going to farmers' markets** on the weekends and stocking up on fresh fruits and vegetables that have been locally grown is a great thing to do. You will be buying produce that is fresher and better tasting with higher nutrition than supermarket produce due to ripening on the tree or vine.

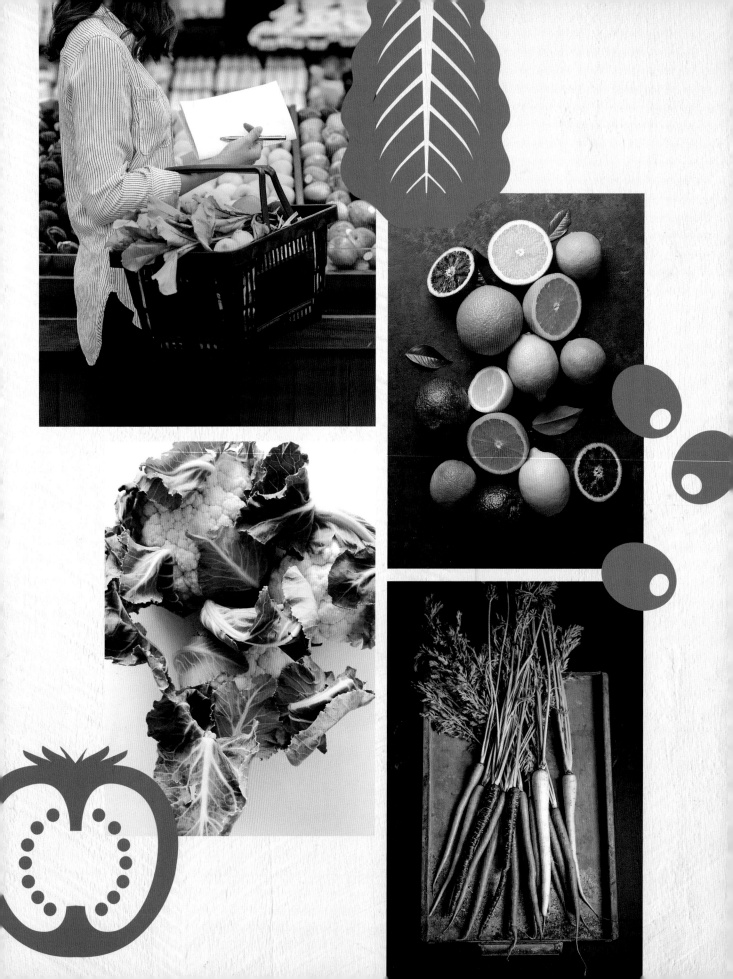

PART 3

Your *heart health* toolkit

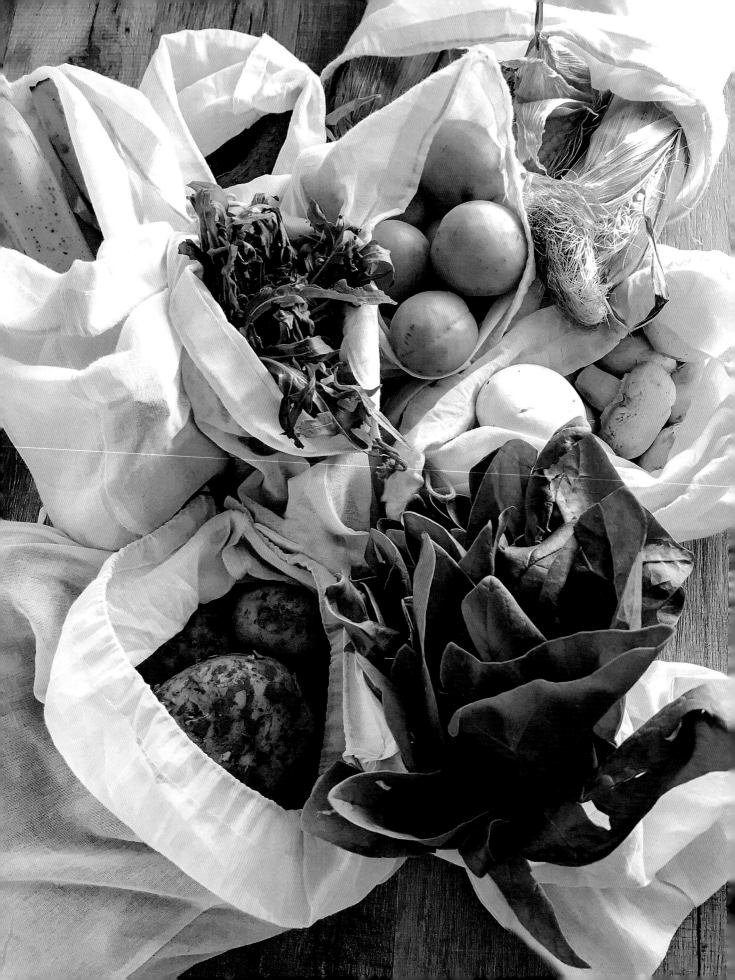

Prepare before you get hungry

Incorporating this Mediterranean diet into your everyday life for heart health is simple if you follow the 10 key principles we talked about on pages 10–11. That's it! It's that easy. Most of us in the Western world are fortunate to have access to an abundant supply of vegetables and fruit, which are now available throughout the year due to sophisticated farming techniques and, of course, the transport of foods from different regions around the world. It is great, though, to focus your cuisine on produce that is grown seasonally and local to you. Not only will these foods be cheaper and better for the environment thanks to their lower carbon footprint, but they'll also taste better as they tend to be fresher and fully ripened in the field – boosting their antioxidant levels.

An important mantra when it comes to Mediterranean cuisine is 'prepare before you get hungry'. Thinking ahead and preparing meals, or at least elements of meals, is important because if you wait until you are ravenously hungry, you are far more likely to reach for an unhealthy snack. (Sound familiar?) Consequently, being prepared in the kitchen is one of the keys to making Mediterranean-style dishes part of your regular routine, as many of them require some degree of preparation. Slower cooking methods such as baking and braising are also common rather than the fast grill or fry and serve approach of many other cuisines.

In this section of the book you will find tips on how to be prepared for enjoying a heart healthy Mediterranean style cuisine, including how to stock your pantry and fridge to ensure you have those key ingredients 'on hand' when you need them. We'll also talk about how to read nutritional panels so you can make informed choices for heart health when shopping. I'm also sharing some weekly meal plans to give you plenty of ideas using examples of heart health weekly menus for weight loss, vegetarians and vegans.

An important mantra when it comes to Mediterranean cuisine is 'prepare before you get hungry'.

Stocking up your pantry, fridge and freezer

At the heart of every Mediterranean kitchen is a cupboard filled with simple staples such as extra-virgin olive oil, tinned tomatoes, herbs and spices, dried fruit and nuts, and legumes/beans. These ingredients form the backbone of most Mediterranean meals, and seasonal produce adds colour and variety throughout the year, as and when it becomes available.

On the following pages, you'll find lists of the ingredients that appear in many of the recipes in this book. You don't have to go out and buy all of these things at once. Instead, a more economical approach is to start replacing ingredients you currently use with Mediterranean-friendly alternatives as they run out.

For fresh produce such as fruit, vegetables, dairy and animal proteins, you can stock your refrigerator with the ingredients you need for the week. Alternatively, if you live within walking distance of the shops, you could walk to the shop most days and buy ingredients on the days you need them and cook them fresh – as is the way in the Mediterranean. This way, you not only take advantage of the specials of the day, but you also get some great exercise.

Take advantage of free time on weekends to cook some favourite dishes for the week ahead. Portion these into containers, then freeze them so you have meals ready and waiting on those nights when you are too tired or arrive home too late to cook. You can also make a few healthy lunches to take to work. Family members, especially hungry teenagers, will appreciate coming home after school or work and thawing a Spicy lentil and sweet potato soup (page 163), Veggie-stuffed capsicums (page 93), Pork and fennel polpette (page 201) or a slice of Harvest pie (page 130)!

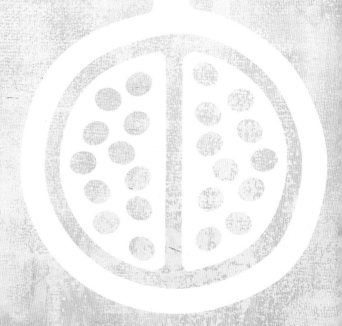

Pantry staples

WHOLEGRAINS, RICE AND PASTA

Wholemeal or gluten-free flour

Polenta

Semolina

Arborio rice

Wild rice

Brown rice

Quinoa

Wholemeal spaghetti

Gluten-free vegetable pasta

Orzo

LEGUMES/BEANS (DRIED OR TINNED)

Chickpeas

Lentils

Cannellini beans

Butter beans

Black beans

Borlotti beans

Four-bean mix

Black-eye peas (usually dried)

Lima beans (usually dried)

TOMATO PRODUCTS

Tinned crushed tomatoes

Tinned tomato purée

Bottled tomato purée/passata

Tomato paste

NUTS AND SEEDS

Walnuts

Almonds

Hazelnuts

Pistachios

Pine nuts

Pumpkin seeds

Sesame seeds

Tahini

Flaxseeds

Chia seeds

DRIED FRUIT

Figs

Dates

Currants

Sultanas

TINNED FISH

Sardines

White anchovies (in jars)

Tuna

Salmon

BEVERAGES

Coffee: espresso style or Greek coffee (if you are game)

Herbal teas

OILS AND VINEGARS

Extra-virgin olive oils

- One for using in cooking and salads
- A lighter variety suitable for making desserts
- A flavoured extra-virgin olive oil such as garlic*, chilli or lemon
- Olives preserved in jars (see page 142)

Balsamic vinegar

White wine vinegar

Red wine vinegar

Apple cider vinegar

Honey

*Garlic-flavoured extra-virgin olive oil can be used in dishes in place of garlic if you or a family member has sensitivities to garlic, e.g. FODMAP intolerance.

DRIED HERBS AND SPICES

Sea salt

Iodised salt

Peppercorns

Ground black pepper

Oregano

Basil

Dill

Parsley

Thyme

Rosemary

Bay leaves

Ground coriander

Fennel seeds

Granulated garlic

Ground turmeric

Ground cinnamon

Ground nutmeg

Cloves: ground and whole

Ground cardamom

Allspice

Ambient storage

FRUIT

Oranges

Mandarins

Grapefruit

Apples

Pears

Lemons

Limes

VEGETABLES

Red onions

Brown onions

Garlic

Potatoes

Sweet potatoes

Tomatoes: cherry, roma and vine-ripened varieties

Fridge

CHEESE AND FERMENTED DAIRY

Feta

Mizithra (whey cheese)

Kefalograviera (Greek gruyere-style)

Goat's cheese

Buffalo mozzarella

Ricotta

Blue cheese

Parmesan

Greek-style yoghurt

Free-range eggs

FRUIT

Strawberries

Cherries

Blueberries

Watermelon

Rockmelon

Grapes

Stone fruits (peaches, plums, apricots)

Figs

Pomegranate

VEGETABLES

Spring onions

Leeks

Celery

Ginger

Beetroot

Capsicums: all colours

Eggplants

Carrots

Cauliflower

Broccoli or broccolini

Green beans

Snap peas

Fennel bulbs

Zucchini

Chillies: red and green

Cucumber

LEAFY GREENS

Cos lettuce

Chicory

Endive

Rocket

Spinach

Mixed mesclun lettuce

Cavolo nero or kale

Wild edible greens

- Dandelion leaves
- Purslane
- Amaranth

FRESH HERBS

Parsley

Dill

Coriander

Basil

Mint

Thyme

Sage

FRESH FISH AND SEAFOOD

Mussels

Squid (calamari)

Octopus

Prawns

Sardines

Whole snapper

Fish fillets (snapper, bream, whiting)

Salmon

Tuna

FRESH FREE-RANGE MEATS (SKIN AND FAT REMOVED)

Chicken

Lamb

Beef and veal

Pork

Kangaroo

Freezer

VEGETABLES

Peas

Broad beans

Green beans

SEAFOOD

Calamari (squid)

Prawns

Fish fillets

MEAT AND PRE-PREPARED MEALS

Mediterranean dishes (leftovers)

Grass-fed beef, lamb or free-range pork (bought in bulk, if possible)

Any cuisine can be made more Mediterranean

To make your diet more Mediterranean and ensure the changes you make are sustainable, it's important to start with small steps that are easy for you to implement. The changes you make to your eating pattern need to be palatable and easy. You do not have to totally transform your diet, give up your favourite dishes or abandon your traditional cultural cuisine to see a health benefit.

Start by making simple changes such as changing the oil you currently use in your kitchen to extra-virgin olive oil and have two meatless days per week. On those days, you can enjoy some of the great-tasting vegetarian dishes in this book, which are full of colourful vegetables, protein-rich legumes and aromatic herbs.

In the diagram and the table that follow, we've shown how some key Mediterranean ingredients can work across a range of ethnic cuisines. With just a few minor modifications, the Mediterranean diet can be flexibly adapted to suit Australians of many backgrounds. We've gone for options that maintain the nutritional benefits, but also take into consideration the availability of ingredients, making it a more environmentally friendly and affordable option for Australians.

Recommendation:

Eat vegetables with every meal

Sub-component of the recommendation:

100 g leafy greens per day

Cretan context examples:

Sow thistle, amaranth, purslane, dandelion, chicory, endive
choose a vegetable that is in season when you can.

Australian context examples:

Spinach, silverbeet, rocket, choy sum, gai lan, bok choy, broccoli, kale
choose a vegetable that is in season when you can.

Adapting favourite dishes to be more Mediterranean

Mediterranean diet guidelines	Greek (Cretan)	Indian	Chinese	Middle Eastern	Western
Guideline: Use extra-virgin olive oil as main fat	Extra-virgin olive oil is used for all cooking and salads.	Swap ghee (clarified butter) for extra-virgin olive oil in curries.	Swap peanut oil and sesame oil for extra-virgin olive oil in stir-fries.	Extra-virgin olive oil is used as the primary fat.	Replace seed oils with extra-virgin olive oil when frying, grilling, baking, stewing and dressing salads.
Guideline: Eat more legumes/beans	**Fasolatha** White beans, onion, garlic, tomato, herbs, extra-virgin olive oil.	**Dhal** Lentils, onion, garlic, tomatoes, ghee. **Swap:** Use extra-virgin olive oil instead of ghee.	**Mapo tofu** Tofu, garlic, spring onion, capsicums, ginger, soy sauce, peanut and/or sesame oils. **Swap:** Use extra-virgin olive oil instead of peanut and/or sesame oil.	**Mujadara** Lentils, onion, spices, extra-virgin olive oil. **Swap:** None. Already Mediterranean!	**Homemade baked beans** Legumes, onion, garlic, tomatoes, vegetable oil. **Swap:** Use extra-virgin olive oil instead of vegetable oil.
Guideline: Eat mainly vegetables and salads with every meal (include leafy greens and tomatoes and fresh herbs)	**Seasonal vegetable bake** (*Briami*) Onion, garlic, eggplant, zucchini, capsicum, potato, chilli, tomatoes, basil, oregano, parsley, extra-virgin olive oil.	**South Indian vegetable curry** Onion, garlic, ginger, cauliflower, sweet potatoes, tomatoes, carrots, spinach, chickpeas, coriander, tomato paste, turmeric, cumin, cayenne pepper, ghee. **Make it more Med:** Use extra-virgin olive oil instead of ghee.	**Vegetable stir-fry** Carrot, broccoli, snow peas, shitake mushrooms, water chestnuts, garlic, ginger, chicken stock, soy sauce, cornflour, rice, peanut oil. **Make it more Med:** Use extra-virgin oil instead of peanut oil, add some cherry tomatoes, use vegetable stock instead of chicken stock and add dried herbs.	**Shakshouka** Onion, garlic, red capsicum, tomatoes, spinach, chickpeas, coriander, parsley, paprika, turmeric, cumin, extra-virgin olive oil. **Make it more Med:** None. It's already Mediterranean!	**Vegetarian Irish stew** Onion, mushrooms, carrots, parsnips, turnips, celery, split peas, vegetable stock, flour, sugar, Vegemite, thyme, rosemary, marjoram. **Make it more Med:** Use extra-virgin olive oil to sauté the vegetables, add fresh tomato, spinach or silverbeet, use cinnamon and nutmeg instead of sugar and Vegemite.

The 4:1 plant to animal ratio on a plate

Rebalance your plate by piling up the vegetables so your meals reflect the Mediterranean plant to animal food ratio of 4:1 to ensure you pack in the nutrition benefits of all the anti-inflammatory and cardioprotective ingredients of the Mediterranean diet. The plates on pages 60 and 61 illustrate what a traditional Mediterranean plate looks like compared to a plate of food that follows a typical Western diet, which has a 1:1 plant to animal food ratio.

To put this into context, think about the serving of animal protein such as meat or chicken that you would normally eat. If is covers half your plate, that portion of meat will be around 250–300 grams. What about the serving of vegetables? If you usually have potatoes with your meat (especially fries) and a small side salad that resembles a garnish rather than a substantial salad, then you haven't achieved this balance.

In contrast, a typical Mediterranean plate will have 70, 80 or 100 grams of animal protein (meat, chicken or fish in that order) and four times as much plant foods – that's about 280–400 grams of vegetables. The non-vegetarian dishes in this cookbook are designed to provide this ratio of 4–5 serves of vegetables for every 1 serving of animal protein. Aim to have at least one of your meals a day look like this (either lunch or dinner) with the other one being a smaller vegetarian meal, such as vegetable soup, stuffed capsicum or cabbage rolls, or perhaps a mixed salad with tinned salmon or tuna. The meal plans on pages 66–73 will help you map out a week of Mediterranean heart healthy eating.

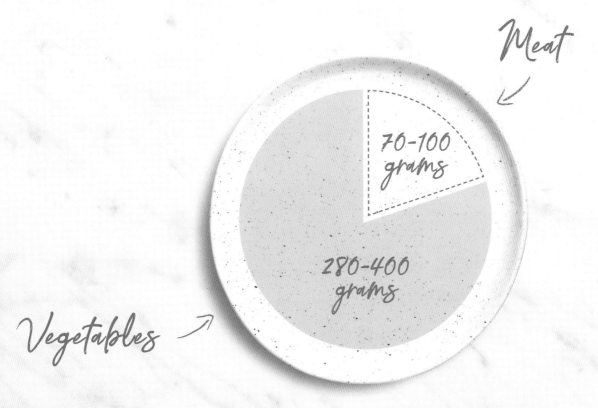

Meat

70–100 grams

280–400 grams

Vegetables

Mediterranean diet

4:1 plant to animal food ratio

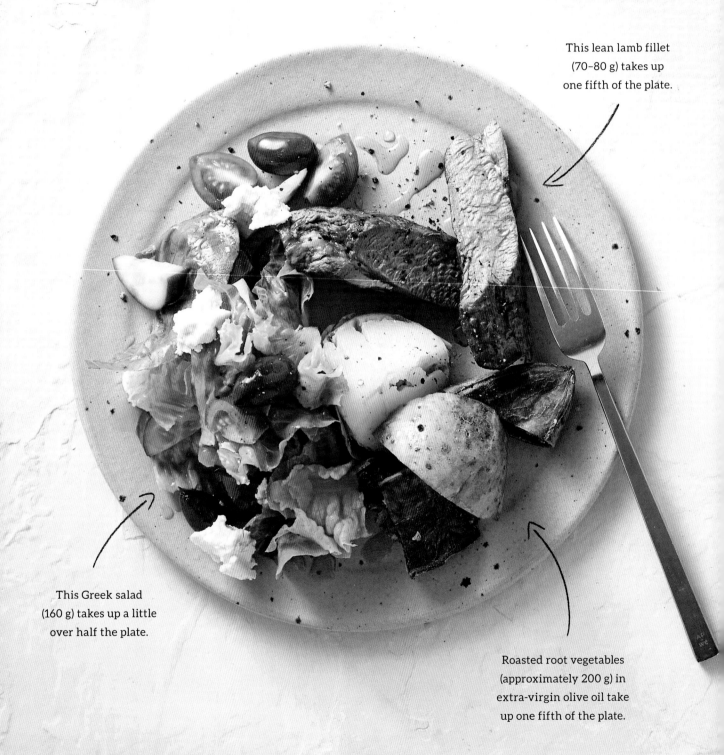

This lean lamb fillet (70–80 g) takes up one fifth of the plate.

This Greek salad (160 g) takes up a little over half the plate.

Roasted root vegetables (approximately 200 g) in extra-virgin olive oil take up one fifth of the plate.

Western diet

1:1 plant to animal food ratio

Just a few green
beans (40 g) garnish
this plate.

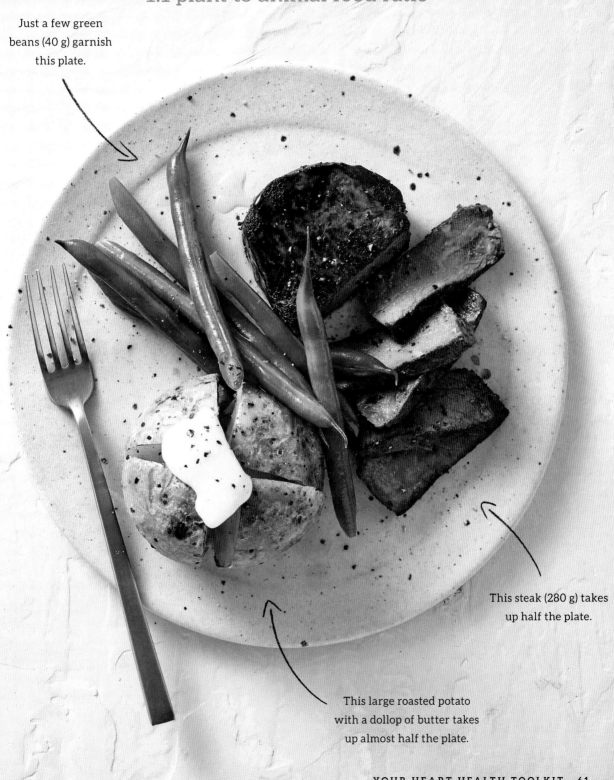

This steak (280 g) takes
up half the plate.

This large roasted potato
with a dollop of butter takes
up almost half the plate.

The Functional Mediterranean Diet Pyramid

Dietary pyramids have been promoted for decades by nutrition authorities across the world. Conceptually, they represent food groups in a way that illustrates an approach to a healthy and balanced diet. Healthy dietary pyramids commonly indicate vegetables and fruit at the base, indicating that those foods should be consumed in larger quantities, followed by wholegrains, then legumes and lean proteins, then dairy near the top – to be consumed in moderate quantities – and fats, oils and sugars to be consumed only occasionally.

The functional Mediterranean pyramid has been developed by an international group of experts in the areas of nutrition, anthropology, sociology and agriculture. It aims to encompass not only the food groups represented in the Mediterranean diet, but also the social and cultural characteristics of the Mediterranean way of life, as inscribed by UNESCO in 2010.

The unique thing about this functional Mediterranean pyramid is its depiction of conviviality: it depicts people sharing meals at the table, cooking seasonal foods together and enjoying group exercise. The elements of this one pyramid pretty much cover a diet and lifestyle prescription for the prevention and management of heart disease.

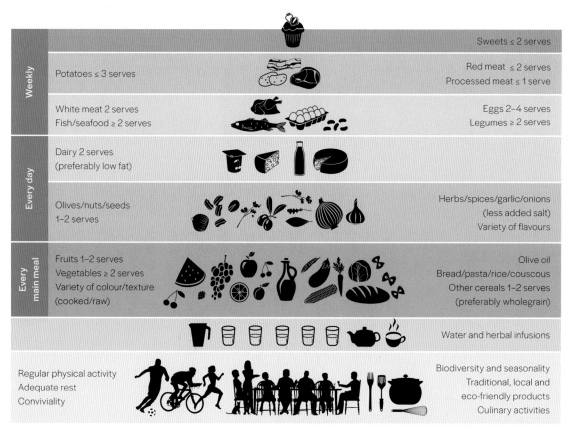

Weekly		Sweets ≤ 2 serves
	Potatoes ≤ 3 serves	Red meat ≤ 2 serves Processed meat ≤ 1 serve
	White meat 2 serves Fish/seafood ≥ 2 serves	Eggs 2–4 serves Legumes ≥ 2 serves
Every day	Dairy 2 serves (preferably low fat)	
	Olives/nuts/seeds 1–2 serves	Herbs/spices/garlic/onions (less added salt) Variety of flavours
Every main meal	Fruits 1–2 serves Vegetables ≥ 2 serves Variety of colour/texture (cooked/raw)	Olive oil Bread/pasta/rice/couscous Other cereals 1–2 serves (preferably wholegrain)
		Water and herbal infusions
	Regular physical activity Adequate rest Conviviality	Biodiversity and seasonality Traditional, local and eco-friendly products Culinary activities

Serving size based on frugality and local habits. Wine in moderation and respecting social beliefs.

Understanding nutritional panels

Ever found yourself gazing at food labels wondering how to decide which product is better for the health of your heart? Aside from the marketing information and health claims made on the label to entice you to try a product, there is a strict requirement on food manufacturers to provide information about every ingredient, especially about any allergens it might contain, such as wheat, nuts or dairy, and where the ingredients are sourced. The ingredients list details everything in a product, from the most concentrated ingredient, which appears first, to the least concentrated. Take care with any foods that include sugar, salt and saturated fats in the first few ingredients.

The nutrition panel on products is another crucial bit of information because it indicates whether that food will help you maintain good health. The panel includes a basic set of nutrients: energy, protein, fats, carbohydrates including sugars, and sodium (or salt). The amounts are shown in two columns: per serve and per 100 grams, which is useful when comparing similar products.

Another very useful element on the nutritional panel is the figure representing the percentage of your daily intake (see note) per serving, as this helps you identify how much of your daily requirements for each nutrient that one serve provides. This is particularly important when assessing if the food is going to be too high in energy (kilojoules or calories) or if it will provide you with a rich source of fibre or antioxidant and anti-inflammatory nutrients such as vitamin C, folate, selenium or omega-3 fats.

Each recipe in this book features a nutrition panel (similar to those on packaged foods) containing information on the energy, protein, fat, carbohydrate, sodium (salt) and fibre content per serving. It also includes attributes of the recipe with respect to whether it is a good source of a specific vitamin or mineral.

Note: What's right for me?

The recommended daily intake (RDI) is the amount of a nutrient (vitamin or mineral) deemed sufficient to meet the needs of nearly all healthy individuals. In fact, only about 10 per cent of the population will have requirements this high; most of us need much less. The RDI provides a buffer, and if you are meeting just under these requirements it does not mean you are deficient. However, if you are consistently only reaching about half these requirements or less, you may be at risk of deficiency in the long term.

In this book, the RDI in the nutrition panels is based on the following:

- Woman aged 30–40 years, 65 kg, office worker with minimal exercise.
- Man aged 30–40 years, 80 kg, office worker with minimal exercise.

You can find out what your specific nutrient requirements are by visiting www.eatforhealth.gov.au.

IDENTIFYING FOOD PRODUCTS FOR HEART HEALTH

When you're out shopping, look at the following categories on the nutritional panel and read the ingredients list to help you assess the heart healthiness of a product:

Energy: Check the kj per serve to see how this stacks up against your daily energy needs. For example, an average 40-year-old woman who is sedentary will need about 8050 kj per day and a 40-year-old man who is sedentary will need about 10,500 kj.

Sugars: Aim to reduce extra sugars by choosing products with less than 15 g of sugars per 100 g. Beware of hidden sugars in products – they'll be labelled in the ingredients list as dextrose, fructose, glucose, golden syrup, honey, malt, maltose, lactose, brown sugar, caster sugar, maple syrup, raw sugar, sucrose.

Fibre: This is an important nutrient when it comes to maintaining a healthy microbiome, and that, in turn leads to a healthier heart. Go for breads, cereals and meals that have a fibre content greater than 3 g per 100 g.

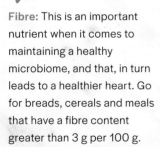

Nutrition Information

Servings per package – 16
Serving size – 30g (⅔ cup)

	Per serve	Per 100g
Energy	432kJ	1441kJ
Protein	2.8g	9.3g
Fat		
Total	0.4g	1.2g
Saturated	0.1g	0.3g
Carbohydrate		
Total	18.9g	62.9g
Sugars	3.5g	11.8g
Fibre	6.4g	21.2g
Sodium	65mg	215mg

Sodium (salt): Sodium is the main mineral in salt (chemical name sodium chloride) and lowering your sodium intake is important if you suffer from high blood pressure. Choose foods that contain less than 400 mg sodium per 100 g. Beware of hidden sources of sodium in the ingredients list in foods such as: baking powder, celery salt, garlic salt, meat/yeast extract, monosodium glutamate (MSG), onion salt, rock salt, sea salt, sodium, sodium ascorbate, sodium bicarbonate, sodium nitrate/nitrite, stock cubes, vegetable salt.

Omega-3 fats: Beneficial long-chain omega-3 fats such as EPA and DHA are found in fish and seafood, and some enriched products. Look for tinned fish with an EPA/DHA content of greater than 90 mg per 100 g for women or 160 mg per 100 g for men to meet daily requirements for a healthy heart. If you already have heart disease, your requirements go up to 400 mg per day.

Saturated fats: Aim for products that have lower levels of saturated fats — less than 3 g of saturated fat per 100 g being the best. Trans fats should be negligible. Saturated fats are often hidden in ingredients lists, and the following foods tend to be very high in saturated fats: animal fat/oil, beef fat, butter, chocolate, milk solids, coconut, coconut oil, milk, cream, copha, cream, ghee, dripping, lard, suet, palm oil, sour cream, vegetable shortening.

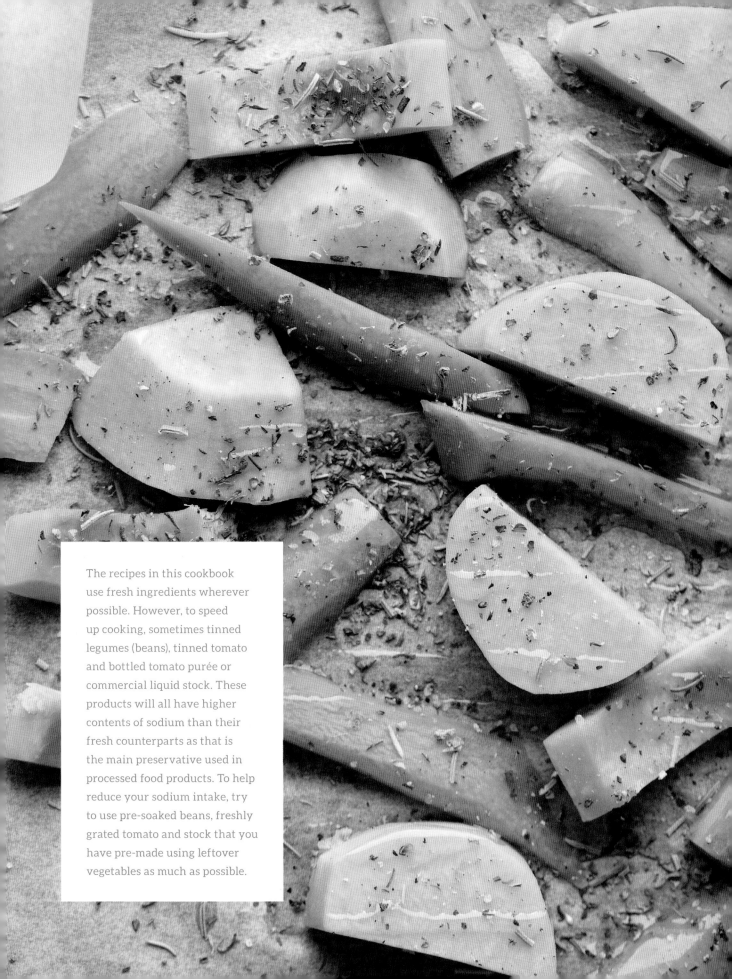

The recipes in this cookbook use fresh ingredients wherever possible. However, to speed up cooking, sometimes tinned legumes (beans), tinned tomato and bottled tomato purée or commercial liquid stock. These products will all have higher contents of sodium than their fresh counterparts as that is the main preservative used in processed food products. To help reduce your sodium intake, try to use pre-soaked beans, freshly grated tomato and stock that you have pre-made using leftover vegetables as much as possible.

Heart Health Guide sample meal plan

This menu is a sample of how you can incorporate my most delicious recipes from *The Heart Health Guide* into your week. It is rich in omega-3 fats, vitamin C, folate and plant antioxidants, and is low in saturated fats scoring high in cardioprotective anti-inflammatory nutrients.

	SUNDAY	MONDAY	TUESDAY	WEDNESDAY
BREAKFAST	Baked eggs with roasted capsicum and chickpeas (page 86) Slice sourdough toast (page 106) Espresso coffee or tea	Horta: sautéed wild greens with feta on sourdough toast (page 89) with a poached egg (optional) Espresso coffee or tea	Greek-style yoghurt (page 78) with blueberries, caramelised crushed pistachios and cinnamon Espresso coffee or tea	Hazelnut butter and tomatoes on sourdough (page 81) Espresso coffee or tea
LUNCH	Chargrilled sardine fillets (page 187) Salad: Zucchini tagliatelle salad with chilli and pistachios (page 134)	Veggie-stuffed capsicums (page 93) Salad: Cos lettuce with crumbled blue cheese	Grilled lean lamb fillets, Chickpea tabbouleh (page 151) and Herb yoghurt (page 205) in wholemeal wrap	Mussels with salsa verde and white wine (page 175) Salad: Seychelles salad (page 145) Slice sourdough bread (page 106)
DINNER	Pork and fennel polpette (page 201) on Skordalia: purple-skinned white sweet potato and garlic mash (page 183) Salad: Citrus and fennel salad (page 152)	Chickpea and rosemary casserole (page 101) with brown rice Salad: Lettuce and cucumber	Marinated tuna steak (page 174) with grilled asparagus and fennel Salad: Greco-Italian salad (page 196)	Quick spaghetti with salmon (page 178) Salad: Cos lettuce, spring onion, fennel
SNACK	Greek-style yoghurt (page 78) with honey, walnuts and cinnamon Orange or mandarin	2–3 dried dates stuffed with almonds Orange or mandarin Healthy Heart pasteli (page 222)	Pear and mandarin 2 dried figs stuffed with walnuts Hazelnut biscuits (page 223)	Greek-style yoghurt (page 78) with fresh berries and nutmeg Mandarin Healthy Heart pasteli (page 222)

NUTRITION COMPOSITION PER DAY:

Energy:	Protein:	Fat:	Carbohydrate:	Fibre:	Vitamin C:	Folate:	B-Carotene:	Long chain omega-3 fats (EPA/DHA):
9060 kj (2157 kcal)	94 g (17% E)	109 g (45% E) Less than 10% E from Saturated Fats	180 g (33% E)	37 g	330 mg	601 µg	4400 µg	850 mg

THURSDAY	FRIDAY	SATURDAY
Greek-style yoghurt (page 78) with Baklava clusters (page 227) and berries or sliced banana Espresso coffee or tea	Mushrooms on toast with pesto and spinach (page 84) with a poached egg (optional) Espresso coffee or tea	Savvas' scrambled eggs with roasted tomatoes, smashed peas and goat's cheese (page 85) Espresso coffee or tea
Spicy green beans (page 98) Salad: Fresh tomato salad (page 141)	Meat and mushroom burger with beetroot, butter bean and yoghurt sauce (page 211)	Healthy heart minestrone (page 164) Salad: Leafy green salad with sugar snap peas and mustard dressing (page 158)
Grilled lean lamb cutlets with roasted pumpkin Salad: Chargrilled cos with pangrattato and grated cheese (page 149)	Kangaroo meatballs and spaghetti (page 192) or swap the pasta for white bean purée Salad: Seychelles salad (page 145)	Marinated pork cutlets with roasted apples (page 212) Salad: Warm broad bean and pea salad (page 137)
Healthy Heart pasteli (page 222) Strawberries Small bunch of red grapes	Greek-style yoghurt (page 78) with pistachios and cinnamon Orange or mandarin	Pistachio baklava (page 226) Watermelon Greek-style yoghurt (page 78) and honey

Heart Health Guide vegetarian meal plan

This cardioprotective menu is designed for vegetarians and is rich in fibre, vitamin C, folate, and plant antioxidants, and is low in saturated fats. *The Heart Health Guide* is full of vegetarian-friendly recipes, and you can find more in 'From the garden' (page 91) and 'Soups and salads' (page 133).

	SUNDAY	MONDAY	TUESDAY	WEDNESDAY
BREAKFAST	Baked eggs with roasted capsicum and chickpeas (page 86) Slice sourdough toast (page 106) Espresso coffee or tea	Greek-style yoghurt (page 78) with Baklava clusters (page 227) and berries or sliced banana Espresso coffee or tea	Horta: sautéed wild greens with feta on sourdough toast (page 89) with a poached egg Espresso coffee or tea	Hazelnut butter and tomatoes on sourdough (page 81) Espresso coffee or tea
LUNCH	Harvest pie (page 130) Salad: Poached pear and fig salad with caramelised walnuts (page 138)	Veggie-stuffed capsicums (page 93) Salad: Cos lettuce with crumbled blue cheese	Spicy green beans (page 98) with wild rice and quinoa Salad: Fresh tomato salad (page 141)	Black-eye pea and vegetable soup (page 160) Slice sourdough bread (page 106)
DINNER	Vegan pastitsio (page 119) Salad: Citrus and fennel salad (page 152)	Lentil pilaf (page 116) and Cauliflower steak with turmeric yoghurt (page 104) Salad: Leafy green salad with sugar snap peas and mustard dressing (page 158)	Vegetarian moussaka with lentil bolognese (page 125) Salad: Greco-Italian salad (page 196)	Cauliflower and broccoli with cannellini beans (page 111) Salad: Cos lettuce, spring onion, fennel
SNACK	Greek-style yoghurt (page 78) with fresh berries Pistachio baklava (page 226) Orange or mandarin Herbal tea	Healthy Heart pasteli (page 222) Lemony yoghurt tart (page 224) Watermelon Herbal Tea	Orange or mandarin 2 dried figs stuffed with walnuts Hazelnut biscuits (page 223) Herbal tea	Greek-style yoghurt (page 78) with fresh berries and nutmeg Orange or mandarin Healthy Heart pasteli (page 222) Herbal tea

NUTRITION COMPOSITION PER DAY:

Energy:	Protein:	Fat:	Carbohydrate:	Fibre:	Vitamin C:	Folate:	B-Carotene:	Long chain omega-3 fats (EPA/DHA):
8430 kj	64 g (13% E)	107 g (47% E) less than 10% E from Saturated fats	171 g (33% E)	41.5 g	317 mg	660 µg	6854 µg	104 mg

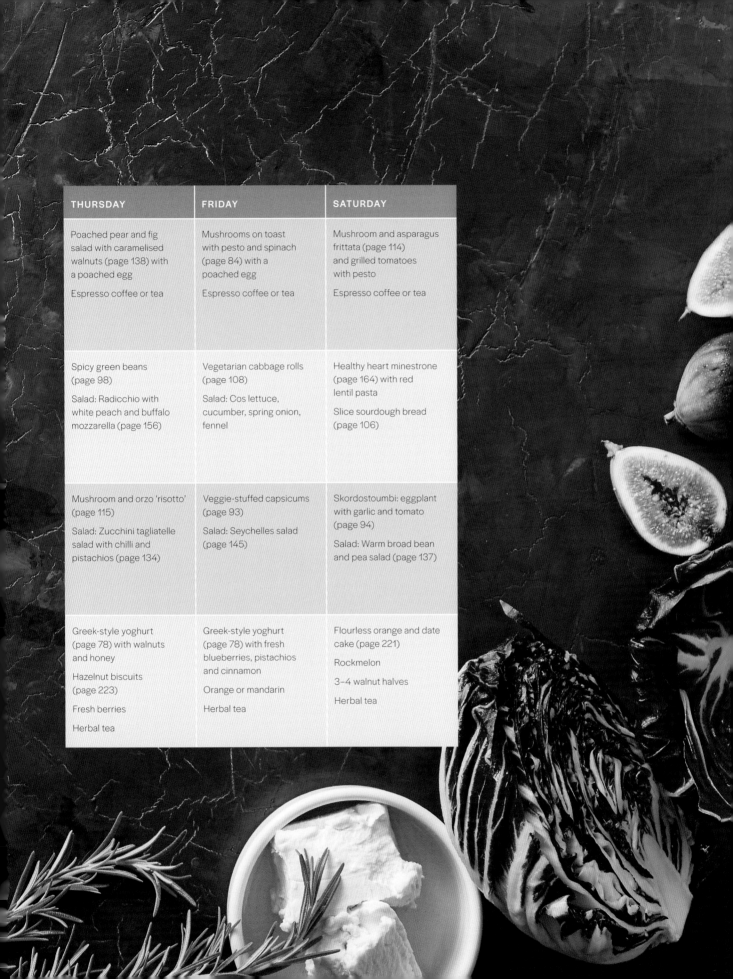

THURSDAY	FRIDAY	SATURDAY
Poached pear and fig salad with caramelised walnuts (page 138) with a poached egg	Mushrooms on toast with pesto and spinach (page 84) with a poached egg	Mushroom and asparagus frittata (page 114) and grilled tomatoes with pesto
Espresso coffee or tea	Espresso coffee or tea	Espresso coffee or tea
Spicy green beans (page 98)	Vegetarian cabbage rolls (page 108)	Healthy heart minestrone (page 164) with red lentil pasta
Salad: Radicchio with white peach and buffalo mozzarella (page 156)	Salad: Cos lettuce, cucumber, spring onion, fennel	Slice sourdough bread (page 106)
Mushroom and orzo 'risotto' (page 115)	Veggie-stuffed capsicums (page 93)	Skordostoumbi: eggplant with garlic and tomato (page 94)
Salad: Zucchini tagliatelle salad with chilli and pistachios (page 134)	Salad: Seychelles salad (page 145)	Salad: Warm broad bean and pea salad (page 137)
Greek-style yoghurt (page 78) with walnuts and honey	Greek-style yoghurt (page 78) with fresh blueberries, pistachios and cinnamon	Flourless orange and date cake (page 221)
Hazelnut biscuits (page 223)	Orange or mandarin	Rockmelon
Fresh berries	Herbal tea	3–4 walnut halves
Herbal tea		Herbal tea

Heart Health Guide vegan meal plan

This healthy heart menu is designed for those who prefer to follow a plant-based diet free of animal foods. It's rich in fibre, vitamin C, folate and plant antioxidants, and shows just how easy it is to supplement with vegan meat and dairy alternatives to ensure adequate protein in your diet.

	SUNDAY	MONDAY	TUESDAY	WEDNESDAY
BREAKFAST	Baked eggs with roasted capsicum and chickpeas (page 86). Replace the eggs with lightly fried firm tofu and replace feta with vegan feta. Slice sourdough bread (page 106) Espresso coffee or tea	Coconut or soy yoghurt with Baklava clusters (page 227) with fresh berries or sliced banana Espresso coffee or tea	Horta: sautéed wild greens with feta on sourdough toast (page 89) Replace the feta with vegan feta and sauté some firm tofu with the greens. Espresso coffee or tea	Hazelnut butter and tomatoes on sourdough (page 81). Omit egg. Espresso coffee or tea
LUNCH	Harvest pie (page 130). Replace ricotta and feta with vegan feta. Salad: Poached pear and fig salad with caramelised walnuts (page 138). Replace the blue cheese with vegan blue cheese. Replace the caramelised walnuts with fresh crushed walnuts.	Veggie-stuffed capsicums (page 93). Replace the feta with vegan feta, if using. Salad: Cos lettuce with crumbled vegan blue cheese	Beef cassoulet (page 215). Replace the beef with cubes of nutmeat and reduce the cooking time to 1 hour. Salad: Fresh tomato salad (page 141). Replace the feta with vegan feta.	Black-eye pea and vegetable soup (page 160) Slice sourdough bread (page 106)
DINNER	Vegan pastitsio (page 119) Salad: Citrus and fennel salad (page 152)	Lentil pilaf (page 116) and Cauliflower steak with turmeric yoghurt (page 104). Replace the Greek-style yoghurt with soy yoghurt. Salad: Leafy green salad	Vegetarian moussaka with lentil bolognese (page 125). Replace the feta with vegan feta and replace the bechamel sauce with bechamel (page 119). Salad: Greco-Italian salad (page 196). Replace the cheese with vegan cheese.	Cauliflower and broccoli with cannellini beans (page 111) Salad: Cos lettuce, spring onion and fennel
SNACK	Coconut or soy yoghurt with berries Pistachio baklava (page 226). Replace honey with maple syrup. Orange or mandarin Herbal tea	Watermelon Healthy Heart pasteli (page 222). Replace honey with maple syrup. 2 tablespoons pistachios Herbal tea	Orange or mandarin 2 dried figs stuffed with walnuts Healthy Heart pasteli (page 222). Replace honey with maple syrup. Herbal tea	Coconut or soy yoghurt with berries and nutmeg Orange or mandarin Healthy Heart pasteli (page 222). Replace honey with maple syrup. Herbal tea

NUTRITION COMPOSITION PER DAY:

Energy:	Protein:	Fat:	Carbohydrate:	Fibre:	Vitamin C:	Folate:	B-Carotene:	Long chain omega-3 fats (EPA/DHA):
8194 kj (1958 kcal)	66 g (14% E)	99.6g (45% E) less than 10% E from Saturated fats	175 g (35% E)	42 g	323 mg	702 µg	5984 µg	25 mg

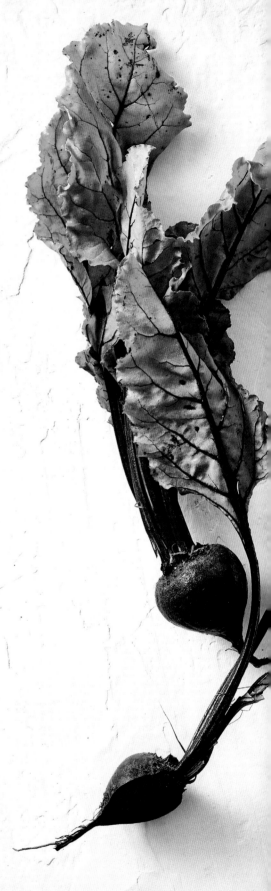

THURSDAY	FRIDAY	SATURDAY
Coconut or soy yoghurt with Baklava clusters (page 227) with fresh berries or sliced banana Espresso coffee or tea	Mushrooms on toast with pesto and spinach (page 84). Omit the egg and replace the parmesan in the pesto with vegan cheese. Espresso coffee or tea	Baked eggs with roasted capsicum and chickpeas (page 86). Replace the eggs with lightly fried firm tofu and replace feta with vegan feta. Slice sourdough bread (page 106) Espresso coffee or tea
Spicy green beans (page 98) Salad: Radicchio with peach and buffalo mozzarella (page 156). Replace the buffalo mozzarella with vegan cheese and replace the caramelised walnuts with fresh crushed walnuts.	Vegetarian cabbage rolls (page 108). In the egg and lemon sauce, replace the egg with aqua faba. Salad: cos lettuce, cucumber, spring onion and fennel	Healthy heart minestrone (page 164) with red lentil pasta Slice sourdough bread (page 106)
Mushroom and orzo 'risotto' (page 115). Replace the butter with dairy-free margarine and replace the parmesan with cashew parmesan cheese. Salad: Zucchini tagliatelle salad with chilli and pistachios (page 134)	Lentil pilaf (page 116) Salad: Seychelles salad (page 145). Replace the cheese with vegan cheese.	Skordostoumbi: eggplant with garlic and tomato (page 94). Replace the cheese with vegan cheese. Salad: Warm broad bean and pea salad (page 137). Replace the cheese with vegan cheese.
Coconut or soy yoghurt with walnuts and drizzle maple syrup. Fresh berries Herbal tea	Coconut or soy yoghurt with blueberries, pistachios and cinnamon Orange or mandarin Herbal tea	Portokalopita: Greek orange cake (page 229). Replace the Greek-style yoghurt with coconut yoghurt. Rockmelon 3–4 walnut halves Herbal tea

Heart Health Guide weight-loss meal plan

This menu is rich omega-3 fats, vitamin C, folate and plant antioxidants, and is low in kilojoules to support weight loss. When following the weight-loss meal plan, try replacing feta with low-fat feta and Greek-style yoghurt with low-fat Greek-style yoghurt.

	SUNDAY	MONDAY	TUESDAY	WEDNESDAY
BREAKFAST	Baked eggs with roasted capsicum and chickpeas (page 86) Espresso coffee or tea	Horta: sautéed wild greens with feta on sourdough toast (page 89) with a poached egg Espresso coffee or tea	Greek-style yoghurt (page 78) with blueberries, caramelised pistachios and cinnamon Espresso coffee or tea	Hazelnut butter and tomatoes on sourdough (page 81) Espresso coffee or tea
LUNCH	Chargrilled sardine fillets (page 187) Salad: Zucchini tagliatelle salad with chilli and pistachios (page 134)	Veggie-stuffed capsicums (page 93) Salad: Cos lettuce with crumbled blue cheese	Grilled lean lamb fillets Salad: Chickpea tabbouleh (page 151) and Herb yoghurt (page 205).	Souzoukakia (page 191) and Herb yoghurt (page 205) Salad: Fresh tomato salad (page 141)
DINNER	Pork and fennel polpette (page 201) on skordalia: purple-skinned sweet potato and garlic mash (page 183) Salad: Citrus and fennel salad (page 152)	Chickpea and rosemary casserole (page 101) with brown rice Salad: Lettuce and cucumber	Marinated tuna steak (page 174) with grilled asparagus and fennel Salad: Greco-Italian salad (page 196)	Tuna and vegetable kebabs with pesto (page 172) Salad: Cos lettuce, spring onion and fennel
SNACK	Greek-style yoghurt (page 78) with walnuts and cinnamon Orange or mandarin Herbal tea	2–3 dried dates stuffed with almonds Orange or mandarin Healthy Heart pasteli (page 222) Herbal tea	Pear and mandarin 2 dried figs stuffed with walnuts Hazelnut biscuits (page 223) Herbal tea	Greek-style yoghurt (page 78) with fresh berries and nutmeg Orange or mandarin Healthy Heart pasteli (page 222) Herbal tea

NUTRITION COMPOSITION PER DAY:

Energy:	Protein:	Fat:	Carbohydrate:	Fibre:	Vitamin C:	Folate:	B-Carotene:	Long chain omega-3 fats (EPA/DHAO:
7160 kj (1700 kcal)	86 g (20% E)	92.5g (47% E) Less than 10% E from Saturated Fats	114 g (26% E)	35 g	403 mg	560 µg	9495 µg	360 mg

THURSDAY	FRIDAY	SATURDAY
Greek-style yoghurt (page 78) with Baklava clusters (page 227) and blueberries Espresso coffee or tea	Mushrooms on toast with pesto and spinach (page 84). Add a poached or boiled egg and omit the sourdough. Espresso coffee or tea	Horta: sautéed wild greens with feta on sourdough toast (page 89). Espresso coffee or tea
Spicy green beans (page 98) Salad: Fresh tomato salad (page 141)	Healthy fish and chips (page 181) Salad: Seychelles salad (page 145)	Healthy heart minestrone (page 164) Salad: Leafy green salad with sugar snap peas and mustard dressing (page 158)
Grilled lean lamb fillets Salad: Chargrilled cos with pangrattato and grated cheese (page 149)	Grilled calamari on cavolo nero pesto (page 168) Salad: Leafy green salad with sugar snap peas and mustard dressing (page 158)	Marinated pork cutlets with roasted apples (page 212) Salad: Warm broad bean and pea salad (page 137)
Healthy Heart pasteli (page 222) Strawberries Small bunch of red grapes Herbal tea	Greek-style yoghurt (page 78) with pistachios and cinnamon Orange or mandarin Herbal tea	A small serve of Pistachio baklava (page 226) Watermelon Herbal tea

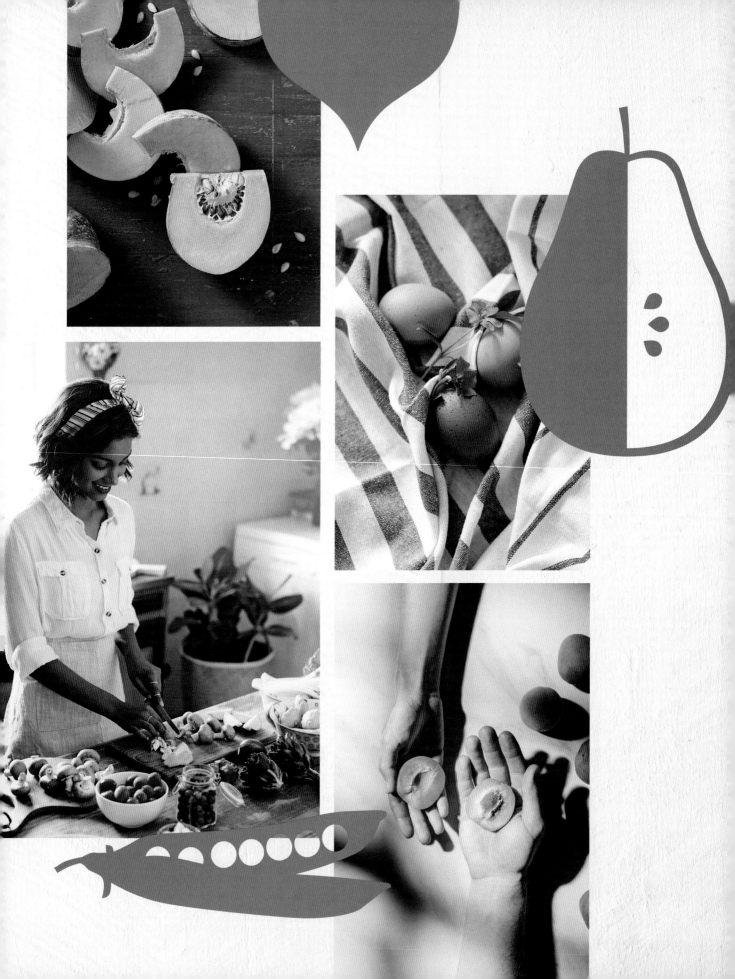

PART 4

Recipes

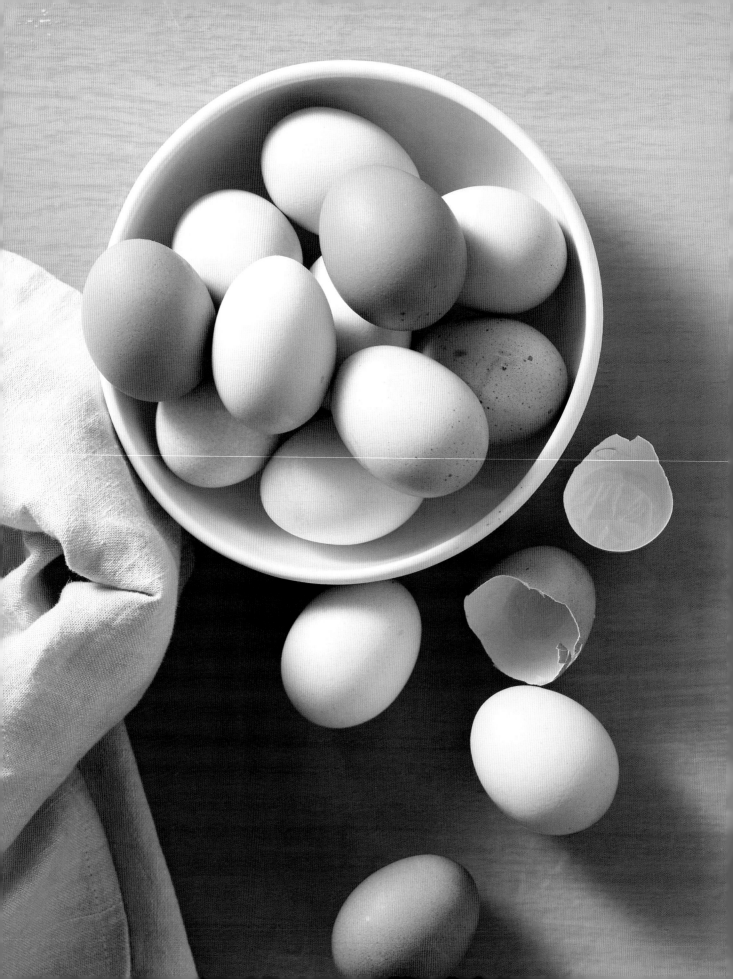

First meal of the day

—

Making *yoghurt*

4 cups (1 litre) full-cream milk (low-fat
milk can be used but the texture of
the yoghurt will be runnier)

3 tablespoons natural yoghurt
with live cultures

Natural yoghurt is a staple food and ingredient in the Mediterranean diet. It's an ideal fermented dairy snack, rich in protein and calcium, and ideal for helping to maintain a healthy microbiome. Greek-style yoghurt has a tart flavour and is thicker than other yoghurts because it is strained. Its health benefits are now known to be due to the probiotics in the yoghurt which are beneficial for gut health.

Step 1: Get your equipment ready: you will need a heavy-based pot, a digital or cooking thermometer to test temperatures and an insulated storage pot (ideally a yoghurt-maker, but you can also use a thermos, or any lidded container wrapped in a warm towel or blanket).

Step 2: Heat treat the milk to destroy undesirable bacteria. To do this, slowly heat the milk in a heavy-based saucepan over a medium heat until it reaches 92°C. Remove the saucepan from the heat and cool the milk down quickly to 35–40°C; you can fill the kitchen sink with cold water and put the saucepan in the sink, but keep an eye on the temperature to ensure it doesn't cool down to lower than 35°C. If it does, warm it up again – cultures need the right temperature.

Step 3: Add the live culture to the warm milk by whisking in the yoghurt.

Step 4: Insulate the mixture by pouring it into a sterilised yoghurt-maker or insulated storage pot (see above) and store in a warm place (the stove if it's being used, or cover with a thick cloth or blanket) for 8 hours, or until the yoghurt sets.

Step 5: Refrigerate and use as required.

TOPPING IDEAS FOR A HEALTHY BREAKFAST OR SNACK:

- Fresh blueberries, chopped dried figs, caramelised pistachios and a drizzle of honey.
- Crushed hazelnuts, sliced fresh figs or chopped dried figs and nutmeg.
- Crushed walnuts with a drizzle of honey and dusting of cinnamon (this is my favourite).

NUTRITION COMPOSITION PER SERVE			
Nutrient	Average Qty per serving	%RDI F	M
Energy	641 kj	8%	6%
Protein	7.6 g	10%	8%
Carbohydrate	13.1 g	5%	4%
Fat	8 g	10%	8%
Sodium	79 mg	4%	4%
Fibre	0 g	0%	0%

High in calcium

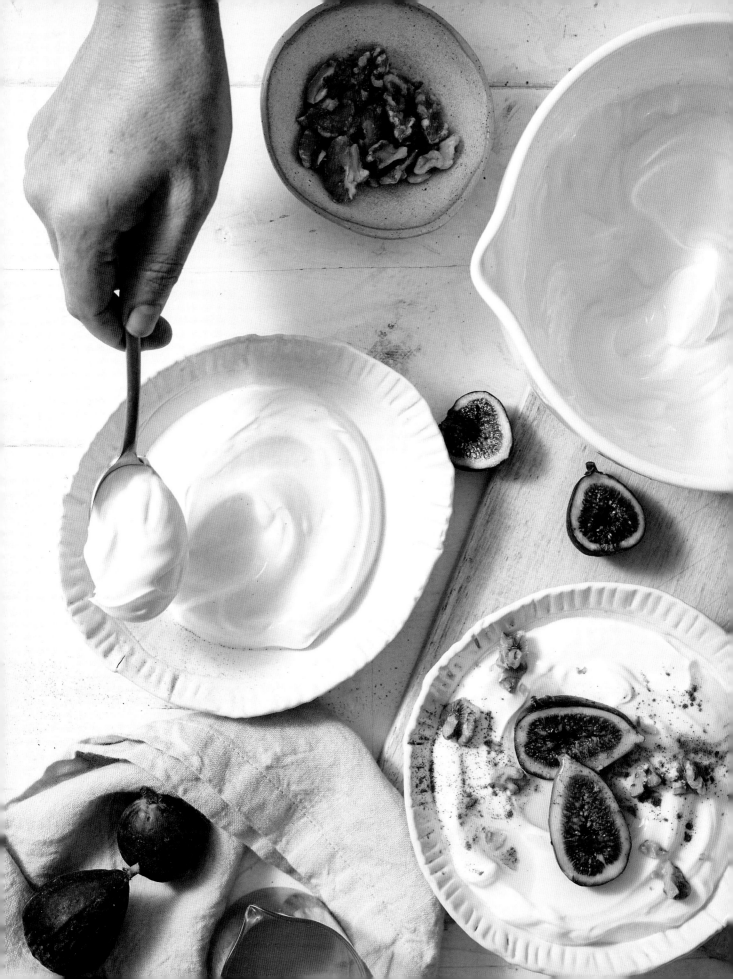

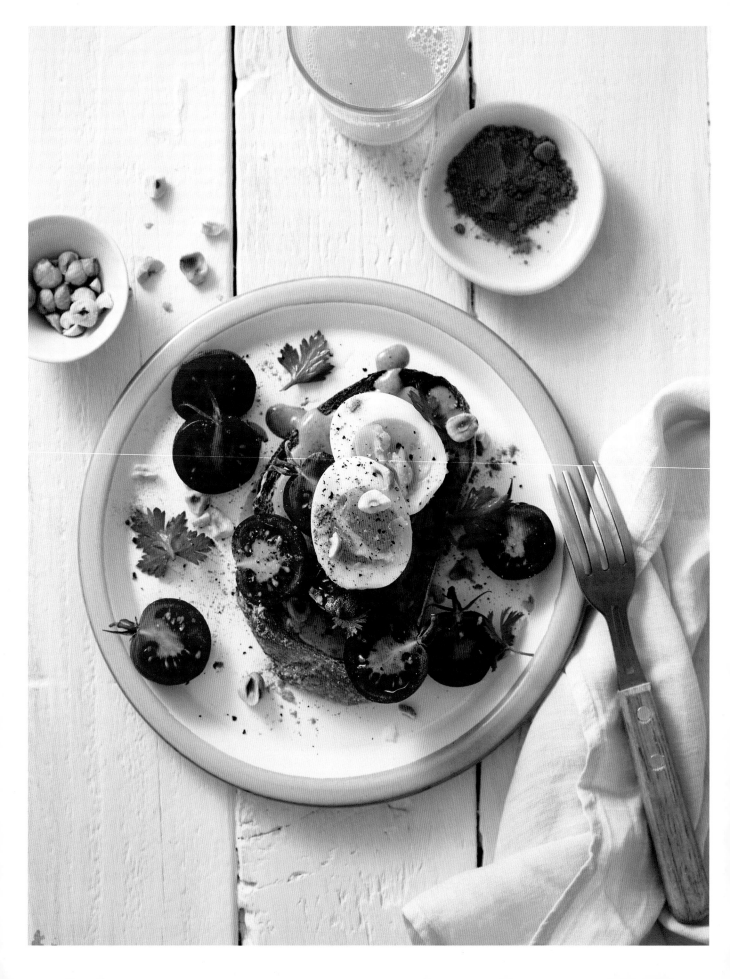

Hazelnut butter and tomatoes
on sourdough

1 tablespoon hazelnut butter

1 thick slice sourdough bread
  (see page 106), toasted

5 cherry tomatoes, halved

1 tablespoon crushed hazelnuts

Sea salt and freshly ground black pepper

1 soft-boiled (or poached) egg, to serve

Ground turmeric, to serve

Fresh herbs, if on hand

This delicious and nutty breakfast toast option is a little different to a usual spread. Hazelnut butter is easily made by simply processing raw hazelnuts in the food processor until creamy. For variation, try almonds, macadamias or roasted peanuts.

Spread the hazelnut butter on the toast. Arrange the cherry tomato halves on top, then sprinkle over the crushed hazelnuts and season with salt and pepper.

To serve, add a soft-boiled (or poached) egg and sprinkle over the turmeric, then garnish with the fresh herbs, if on hand.

NUTRITION COMPOSITION PER SERVE			
Nutrient	Average Qty per serving	%RDI F	M
Energy	1850 kj	22%	18%
Protein	15.6 g	21%	17%
Carbohydrate	26 g	10%	8%
Fat	29 g	36%	30%
Sodium	385 mg	19%	19%
Fibre	5.6 g	20%	15%

High in selenium

Scrambled eggs with roasted tomato and fried potato

COOKING
40 MINUTES

SERVES
4

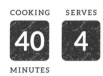

2–3 roma tomatoes, chopped

Extra-virgin olive oil

Sea salt and freshly ground black pepper

2 large potatoes, peeled and diced

1 red onion, finely chopped

6 eggs

Optional: chilli flakes or finely sliced
  red chilli

50 g feta, crumbled

Fresh herbs, if on hand

If you've grown up in a Greek household you will have certainly had a dish called patates me avga – put simply, it's a chip omelette. I've added roasted tomato to add some flavour and boost those antioxidants, of course.

Preheat the oven to 200°C. Line a baking tray with baking paper and arrange the tomato around the tray. Drizzle over the olive oil and sprinkle with salt, then roast for 20 minutes.

Pour enough olive oil to come a third of the way up the side of a large heavy-based frying pan, then place over a medium–high heat until a piece of bread dropped in the oil turns golden. Carefully lower the diced potato into the oil using a slotted spoon, fry until golden, then remove with the slotted spoon and transfer to a plate lined with kitchen paper to drain.

Carefully drain the oil from the frying pan, then return to a medium heat and sauté the onion until softened and translucent. Add the eggs and stir with a fork. When the egg has almost set, add the roasted tomato and fried potato and stir through.

Add a pinch of chilli flakes or chilli slices (if using) to the scrambled eggs. Season with salt and pepper, crumble over the feta, garnish with the fresh herbs, if on hand, and serve right away.

TIP

Extra-virgin olive oil is more expensive than many other oils, so you can make it go further: after using it for frying, allow the oil to cool, then carefully strain it into a clean jar or other container. You can re-use that oil another three or four times for frying, especially if you have only fried potatoes in it.

NUTRITION COMPOSITION PER SERVE

Nutrient	Average Qty per serving	%RDI F	M
Energy	1192 kj	14%	12%
Protein	15 g	21%	17%
Carbohydrate	12.4 g	5%	4%
Fat	18.6 g	23%	19%
Sodium	346 mg	17%	17%
Fibre	3.4 g	12%	9%

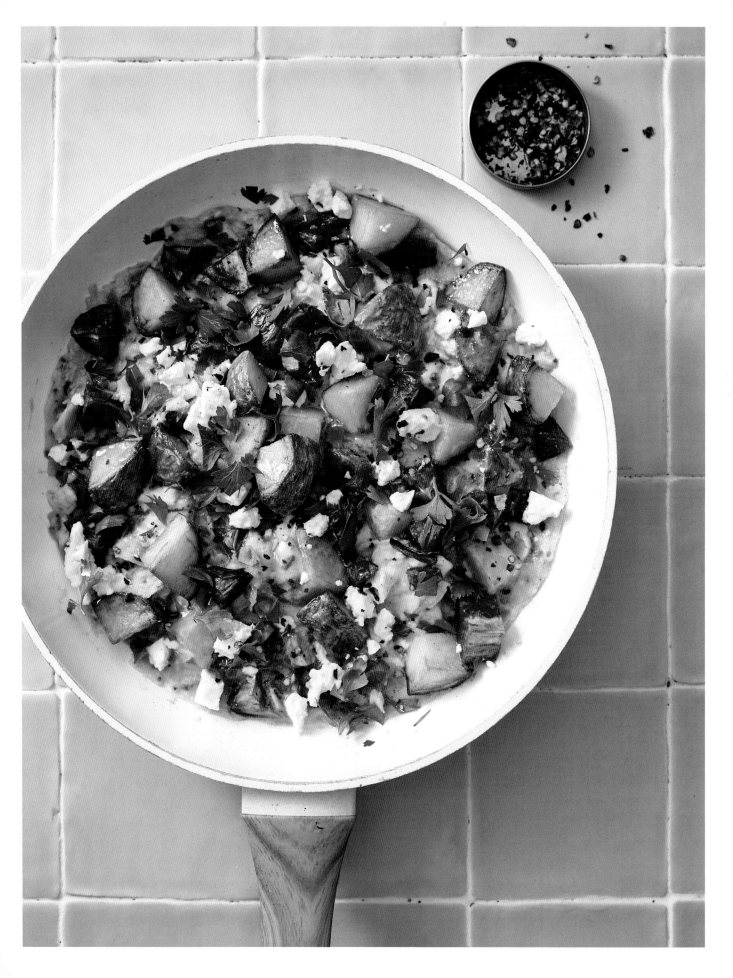

Mushrooms on toast with pesto and spinach

COOKING

10

MINUTES

SERVES

1

1 cup (80 g) button mushrooms, cleaned
and left whole or halved

1 tablespoon Traditional basil pesto
(see below)

Optional: 1 egg, poached

½ cup (25 g) baby spinach leaves

1 thick slice sourdough rye bread, toasted

Sea salt and freshly ground black pepper

Fresh herbs, if on hand

TRADITIONAL BASIL PESTO

1 cup (60 g) basil leaves

30 g pine nuts, toasted

1 garlic clove, peeled

45 g Parmigiano-Reggiano or parmesan

¼ teaspoon freshly ground black pepper

¼ cup (60 ml) extra-virgin olive oil

This Mediterranean-style mushrooms on toast is a popular breakfast option on most cafe menus these days. Vary the flavours by adding a salty Greek cheese such as kefalograviera to the basil pesto or swapping the basil for a mixture of Thai basil and coriander.

Begin by making the pesto: add all the ingredients except the olive oil to a food processor and purée. Gradually add the olive oil and continue to blend until smooth. Set aside.

Sauté the mushrooms over a high heat in a non-stick frying pan for a few minutes until they begin to soften and turn golden. Add the tablespoon of pesto and fry for a few more minutes. If desired, poach the egg while the mushrooms cook.

Add the baby spinach to the mushrooms and toss through, then arrange on top of the toast. Top with the poached egg (if using) and season with salt and pepper. Garnish with the fresh herbs, if on hand, and serve.

NUTRITION COMPOSITION PER SERVE			
Nutrient	Average Qty per serving	%RDI F	M
Energy	655 kj	8%	6%
Protein	6.8 g	9%	8%
Carbohydrate	15.1 g	6%	5%
Fat	7 g	9%	7%
Sodium	192 mg	10%	10%
Fibre	2 g	7%	5%

Savvas' *scrambled eggs* with roasted tomato, smashed peas and goat's cheese

COOKING
20 MINUTES

SERVES
1

5 cherry tomatoes

Extra-virgin olive oil

Chilli flakes (see intro)

Mixed dried herbs

Sea salt and freshly ground black pepper

½ cup (70 g) frozen peas

3 mint sprigs, leaves picked

2 eggs

1 tablespoon crème fraîche

1 teaspoon finely chopped chives

1 thick slice sourdough bread (see page 106), toasted

20 g fresh goat's cheese, crumbled

Fresh herbs, if on hand

A favourite breakfast at my house is my husband Savvas' scrambled eggs – creamy with lots of chilli and chives. My family loves chilli so you will see most traditional Mediterranean recipes have been 'pimped-up' with chilli, which is optional if you don't fancy spicy foods.

Preheat the oven to 180°C. Line a baking tray with baking paper and place the cherry tomatoes on the tray. Drizzle over some olive oil and sprinkle over a pinch of chilli flakes, dried herbs and season with salt and pepper to taste. Roast for 20 minutes.

To make the smashed peas, boil the frozen peas for a few minutes, then drain well and add to a food processor with the mint leaves and 1 teaspoon of olive oil. Season with salt, pepper and a pinch of chilli flakes and pulse so they are smooth, but still have some texture to them. Set aside.

A few minutes before you are ready to serve, make the scrambled eggs. For creamy eggs, crack the eggs into a heavy-based saucepan, season with salt and pepper and a pinch of chilli flakes and place on a low heat. Stir gently with a whisk. Gradually add the crème fraîche and keep stirring until the eggs are set. Stir in the chives, then remove from the heat.

To serve, spread the smashed peas on the toast, then spoon on the scrambled eggs. Top with the roasted tomatoes, crumble over the goat's cheese and garnish with the fresh herbs, if on hand.

NUTRITION COMPOSITION PER SERVE			
Nutrient	Average Qty per serving	%RDI F	M
Energy	2682 kj	33%	26%
Protein	27.8 g	38%	31%
Carbohydrate	46.5 g	19%	15%
Fat	36.5 g	46%	37%
Sodium	492 mg	25%	25%
Fibre	8.3 g	30%	22%

High in fibre

Baked eggs with roasted capsicum and chickpeas

COOKING **25** MINUTES

SERVES **4**

¼ cup (60 ml) extra-virgin olive oil

1 small red onion, finely chopped

2 x 400 g tins chickpeas, drained and rinsed

1 cup (250 ml) puréed tomato

1 cup (250 ml) boiling water

4–6 baby capsicums, roasted, deseeded and cut into strips, or 1 x 330 g jar roasted peppers, drained

¼ teaspoon ground nutmeg

Sea salt and freshly ground black pepper

Optional: chilli flakes or finely sliced small red chilli and mixed dried herbs

4 eggs

20 g feta, crumbled

Fresh herbs, if on hand

This spicy Greek-style shakshuka is made with chickpeas to boost the plant protein and fibre. Adding crumbled feta is a nice touch.

Heat the olive oil in a large heavy-based frying pan over a medium heat and sauté the onion until softened and translucent, then add the chickpeas and cook for a further 5 minutes.

Add the puréed tomato and boiling water to the frying pan, stir, then add the roasted capsicum and simmer for 5–10 minutes. Add the nutmeg and season with salt, pepper, chilli flakes or chilli and/or dried herbs (if using).

One at a time, crack the eggs into a small glass. Use a spoon to make cavities in the chickpea mixture. Carefully place an egg in each hole and simmer slowly until the eggs are cooked. To quickly set the eggs, you can place a lid on the frying pan (best if it's a glass lid so you can see how the eggs are cooking). If you are using an oven-safe frying pan, this last step can be done in an oven preheated to 180°C for about 5 minutes, or until the eggs are cooked to your liking.

Garnish with the feta and fresh herbs, if on hand, before taking to the table so everyone can serve themselves.

NUTRITION COMPOSITION PER SERVE			
Nutrient	Average Qty per serving	%RDI F	M
Energy	1683 kj	20%	16%
Protein	18.2 g	24%	20%
Carbohydrate	25.1 g	10%	8%
Fat	22.6 g	27%	22%
Sodium	554 mg	28%	28%
Fibre	11 g	39%	29%

High in fibre, vitamin C and b-carotene

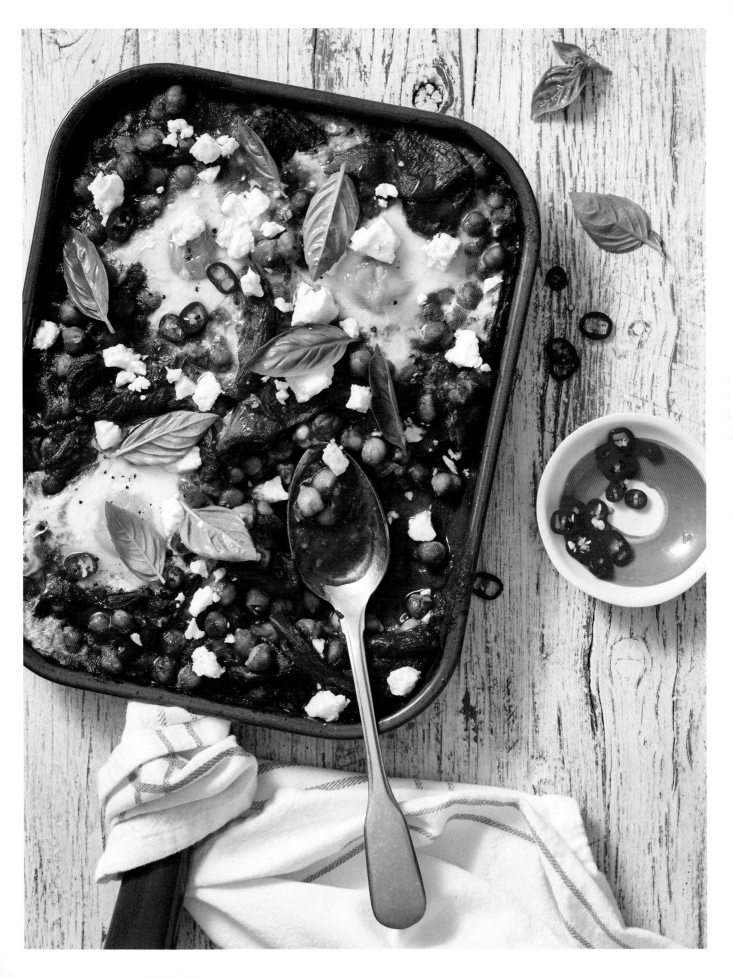

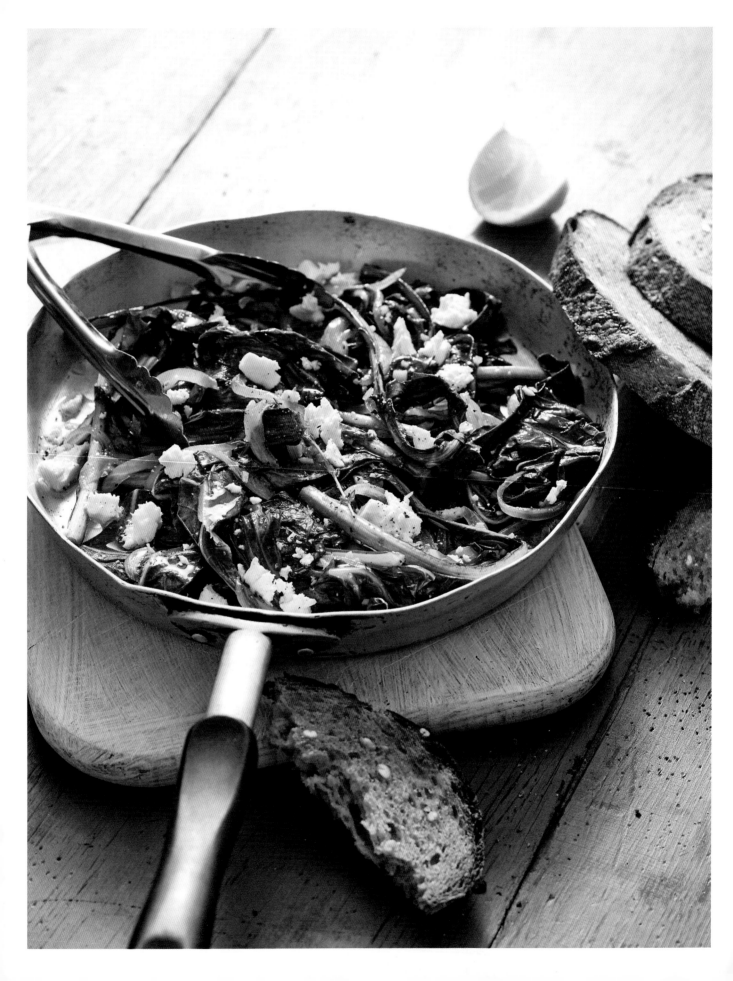

Horta: sautéed wild greens with feta and sourdough toast

1 tablespoon extra-virgin olive oil

1 small red onion, finely sliced

1 garlic clove, finely sliced

1 cup bitter greens, such as chicory, endive, silverbeet, rainbow chard or kale, washed and roughly chopped (remove stems if using kale)

3 thyme sprigs, leaves picked

Sea salt and freshly ground black pepper

1 thick slice sourdough bread (see page 106), toasted

20 g feta, crumbled

Fresh herbs and lemon wedges, if on hand

Wild edible greens – or horta in Greek – are a rich source of antioxidant and anti-inflammatory nutrients. The best way to enjoy these bitter greens is to sauté them with extra-virgin olive oil and dress with lemon juice.

Heat the olive oil in a large heavy-based frying pan over a medium heat and sauté the onion until softened and translucent. Add the garlic and sauté for a few more minutes, taking care not to burn the garlic.

Add the greens and continue to cook until they have wilted – tougher greens like silverbeet and kale will need more cooking. Add the thyme and season with salt and pepper to taste.

Layer the cooked wild greens on the sourdough toast. Crumble over the feta and garnish with the fresh herbs and lemon wedges, if on hand.

NUTRITION COMPOSITION PER SERVE			
Nutrient	Average Qty per serving	%RDI F	M
Energy	1492 kj	18%	15%
Protein	11.7 g	16%	13%
Carbohydrate	19.6 g	8%	6%
Fat	24.1 g	30%	25%
Sodium	577 mg	29%	29%
Fibre	7.9 g	28%	21%

High in fibre and folate

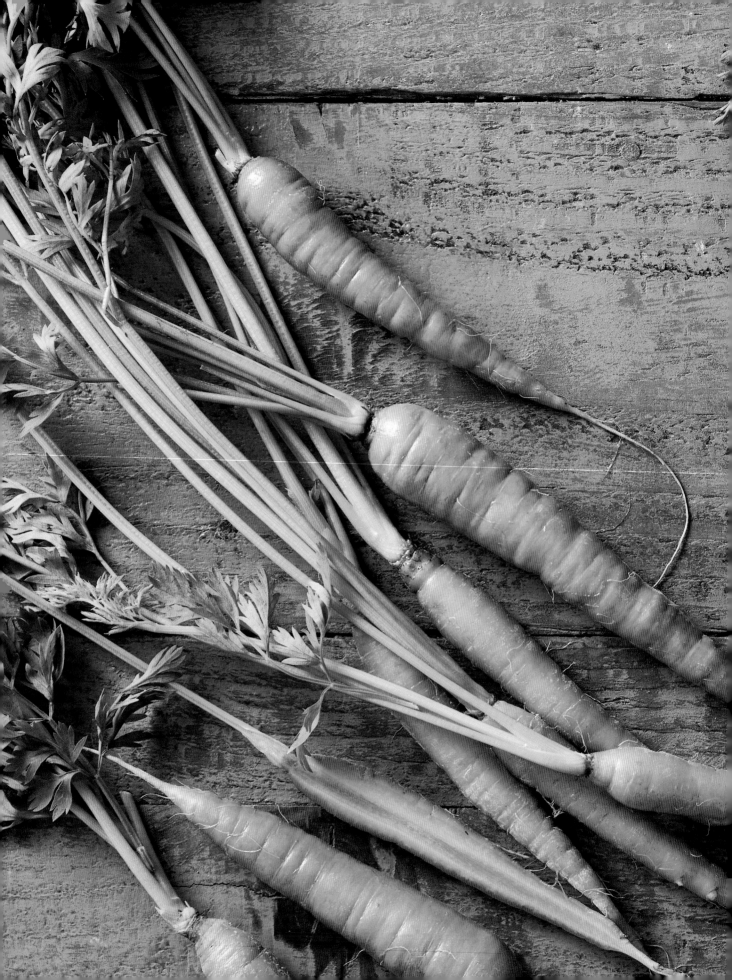

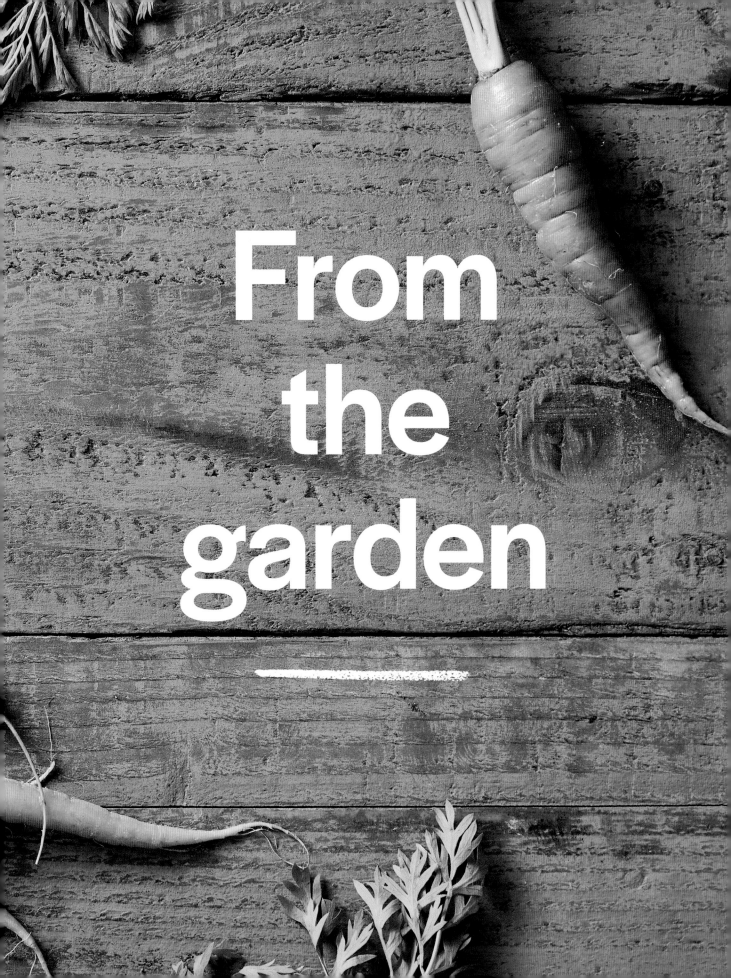

From the garden

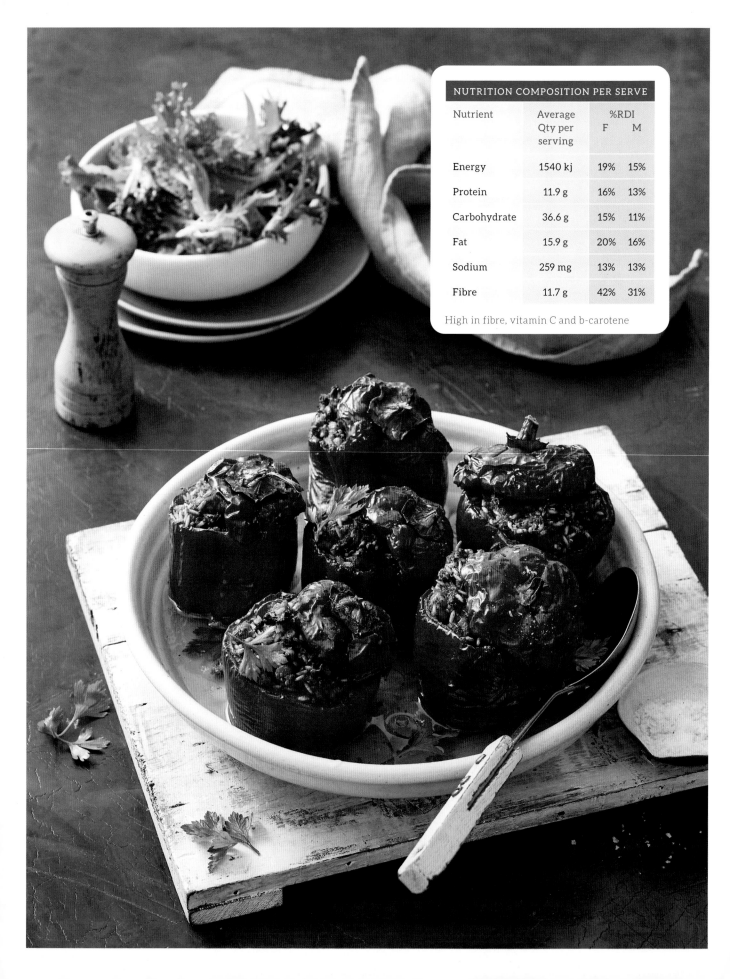

NUTRITION COMPOSITION PER SERVE			
Nutrient	Average Qty per serving	%RDI F	M
Energy	1540 kj	19%	15%
Protein	11.9 g	16%	13%
Carbohydrate	36.6 g	15%	11%
Fat	15.9 g	20%	16%
Sodium	259 mg	13%	13%
Fibre	11.7 g	42%	31%

High in fibre, vitamin C and b-carotene

Veggie-stuffed capsicums

6 capsicums (see intro)

¼ cup (60 ml) extra-virgin olive oil, plus
    ¼ cup (60 ml) for baking

1 small red onion, finely diced

2 garlic cloves, finely diced

1 small red chilli, halved, deseeded
    and finely chopped

¼ fennel bulb, finely diced

Optional: diced Swiss brown mushrooms

200 g black-eyed peas, soaked overnight,
    drained and rinsed, or 1 x 400 g tin,
    drained and rinsed

¾ cup (150 g) mixture of brown rice
    and quinoa (see note)

Optional: ½ cup (125 ml) dry white wine

4 tomatoes, skinned and puréed, or 1 cup
    (250 ml) puréed tomato

2 cups (500 ml) boiling water, plus ½ cup
    (125 ml) for baking

1 tablespoon finely chopped flat-leaf
    parsley, plus extra leaves to serve

Sea salt and freshly ground black pepper

Leafy green salad, to serve

Optional: feta, crumbled, to serve

Stuffed capsicums make the ideal filling lunch; they can be eaten hot or cold and also freeze well for last-minute meals. The plant protein from the beans and fibre from the brown rice and quinoa make these very satiating. Choose wide capsicums as they are easier to stuff. Any colour goes, mix it up.

Carefully cut around the stem of each capsicum and remove the top. Keep these to use as 'lids' for the capsicums during cooking. Discard the seeds.

Heat the olive oil in a large heavy-based saucepan over a medium heat and sauté the onion until softened and translucent. Add the garlic, chilli, fennel and mushroom (if using) and continue to cook for a few minutes until the fennel softens. Add the black-eyed peas and rice and quinoa mixture, then stir in the white wine (if using). Cook for a few minutes, or until most of the alcohol has evaporated.

Add the puréed tomato and 2 cups of boiling water, and simmer for around 10 minutes, or until the rice softens. If the rice is still crunchy, add another cup of boiling water. Stir in the parsley and season with salt and pepper to taste. Remove the mixture from the heat and allow to cool for 10–15 minutes.

Stand the capsicums in a deep baking dish, tops facing up, and carefully divide the cooled mixture between the capsicums, filling each one to the top. Put their lids on.

Pour the ¼ cup of olive oil and ½ cup of boiling water around the capsicums and bake for 45 minutes, checking that the capsicums aren't burning and adding a splash more boiling water if necessary (if the pan is dry).

Allow the capsicums to cool a little, then scatter over the flat-leaf parsley leaves and serve with a leafy salad and a small serve of feta (if using).

NOTE

You can buy brown rice and quinoa mixtures in microwaveable sachets, but if you're making your own, use 100 g of brown rice and 50 g of quinoa.

Skordostoumbi: eggplant with garlic and tomato

½ cup (125 ml) extra-virgin olive oil

3 eggplants, sliced into thick rounds

3 garlic cloves, crushed

1 x 400 g tin chopped tomatoes

1 cup (250 ml) puréed tomato

Optional: ½ cup (125 ml) dry white wine

¼ teaspoon oregano leaves

Sea salt and freshly ground black pepper

50 g feta

Fresh herbs, if on hand

Polenta or brown rice, to serve

If you love eggplants and garlic, then this is the dish for you. Skordostoumbi is a classic vegetarian dish from the island of Zakynthos and resembles eggplant parmigiana – not surprising, as this Greek island has a strong Italian influence.

Heat ¼ cup (60 ml) of the olive oil in a large non-stick frying pan over a medium–low heat and gently fry the eggplant in batches until lightly browned on both sides, then set aside.

Heat the remaining olive oil in a large non-stick casserole dish, and gently sauté the garlic for a minute or two, making sure not to let the garlic burn. Add the tinned tomatoes, puréed tomato and wine (if using) and simmer for 10 minutes.

Add the eggplant and oregano to the dish and season with salt and pepper. Simmer for 10 minutes without stirring. Remove from the heat, crumble the feta on top and garnish with the fresh herbs, if on hand. Serve with some Creamy polenta (see page 198) or steamed brown rice.

NUTRITION COMPOSITION PER SERVE			
Nutrient	Average Qty per serving	%RDI F	M
Energy	1812 kj	22%	18%
Protein	8.9 g	12%	10%
Carbohydrate	17.5 g	7%	5%
Fat	13.7 g	17%	14%
Sodium	406 mg	20%	20%
Fibre	13.2 g	47%	35%

High in fibre

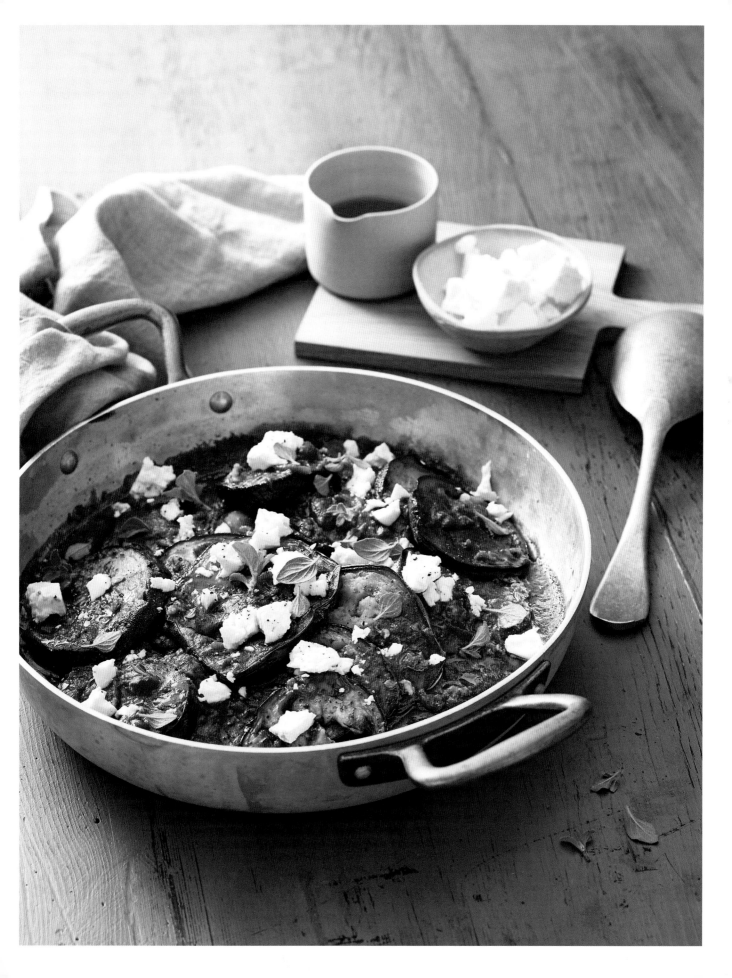

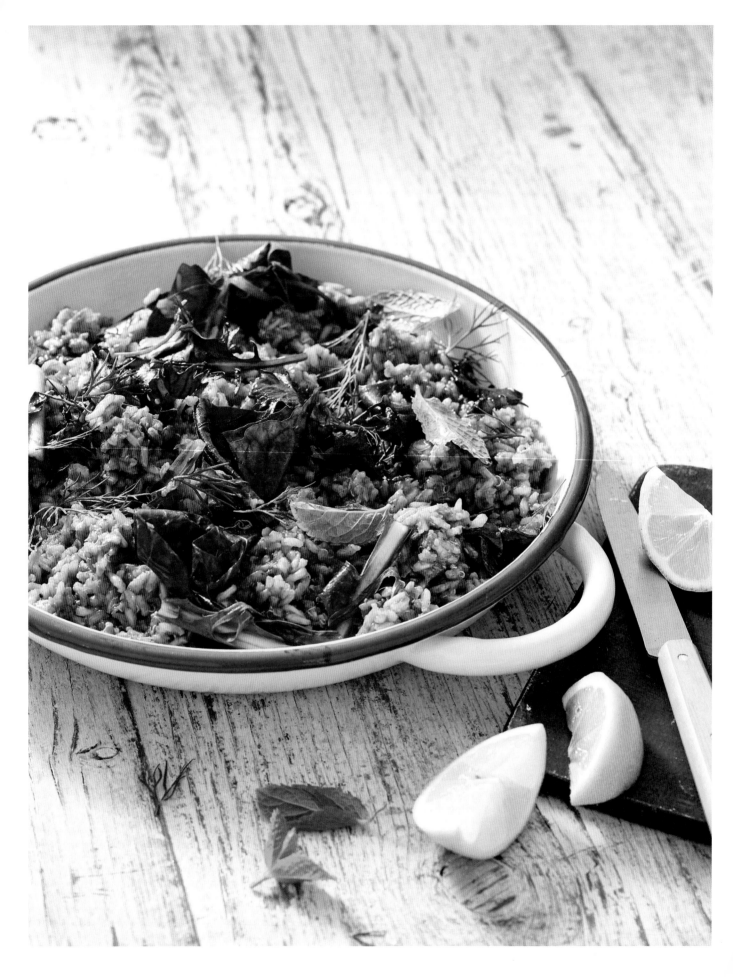

Brown rice and quinoa with greens

2 tablespoons extra-virgin olive oil

1 small red onion, finely diced

1 garlic clove, finely diced

1 small red chilli, halved, deseeded
and finely sliced

180 g brown rice

2 tablespoons quinoa, rinsed

100 g bitter greens, such as beet tops,
collard, kale or Chinese greens,
roughly chopped

1 cup (250 ml) puréed tomato (or grated
fresh tomato, see tip)

2 cups (500 ml) water

Sea salt and freshly ground black pepper

Fresh herbs and lemon wedges, if on hand

This pilaf-style dish is a variation on the traditional spanakorizo (spinach and rice), using brown rice and quinoa instead of white rice to boost fibre and plant omega-3 fats, and mixed bitter greens instead of spinach. It can be served as a side or as a light lunch or dinner.

Heat the olive oil in a saucepan over a medium heat and sauté the onion for a few minutes. Add the garlic and chilli and cook for a few minutes, then add the rice and quinoa and sauté until the rice starts to look a little translucent.

Add the chopped greens and continue to cook until wilted, then add the puréed tomato and water and season with salt and pepper to taste. Turn down the heat to low and cook with the lid on for 30 minutes, or until the rice is cooked.

Garnish with the fresh herbs and lemon wedges, if on hand.

TIP

Grating tomatoes Adding beautiful ripe tomatoes to dishes not only improves the flavour of the dish, it also guarantees there are no additives such as salt and sugar, which you need to watch out for when buying puréed tomato in tins or bottles. To use fresh tomatoes, halve them, then carefully grate the cut side of each half.

NUTRITION COMPOSITION PER SERVE			
Nutrient	Average Qty per serving	%RDI F	M
Energy	1356 kj	16%	13%
Protein	7.5 g	10%	8%
Carbohydrate	44.1 g	18%	14%
Fat	11.5 g	14%	12%
Sodium	173 mg	9%	9%
Fibre	6 g	21%	16%

High in b-carotene

Spicy *green beans*

COOKING
30
MINUTES

SERVES
4

¼ cup (60 ml) extra-virgin olive oil

1 onion, finely chopped

1 small red chilli, halved, deseeded
and finely sliced

500 g green beans, trimmed and halved

1 purple sweet potato, peeled and
thickly sliced

1 orange sweet potato, peeled and
thickly sliced

1 cup (250 ml) puréed tomato

2–3 flat-leaf parsley sprigs, finely chopped

2 garlic cloves, crushed

Sea salt and freshly ground black pepper

4 cups (1 litre) boiling water

1 x 400 g tin borlotti beans, drained
and rinsed

Dried oregano

Fresh herbs, if on hand

Fassoulakia pikantika is a dish best prepared when green runner beans are in season, and are fresh and crisp. The addition of borlotti beans and sweet potato make this a substantial vegetarian dish.

Heat the olive oil in a large heavy-based saucepan over a medium heat and sauté the onion and chilli for 1–2 minutes.

Add the green beans to the pan and cook for 5 minutes. Add the sweet potato and sauté for a few seconds, then add the tomato, parsley and garlic. Season with salt and pepper to taste, and stir well.

Add enough boiling water to cover the vegetables and simmer for 5 minutes. Add the borlotti beans and stir, then simmer for a further 10 minutes, or until the sweet potato is cooked. Add a few pinches of oregano, then taste and adjust the seasonings if necessary before serving. Garnish with the fresh herbs, if on hand.

TIP

If you have time, for better texture and flavour it is best to soak dried borlotti beans overnight and use those instead of tinned. If using this way, add the soaked borlotti beans at the start with the green beans.

NUTRITION COMPOSITION PER SERVE			
Nutrient	Average Qty per serving	%RDI F	M
Energy	1357 kj	16%	13%
Protein	9.6 g	13%	11%
Carbohydrate	30 g	12%	9%
Fat	15.6 g	20%	16%
Sodium	387 mg	19%	19%
Fibre	12.8 g	46%	34%

High in fibre

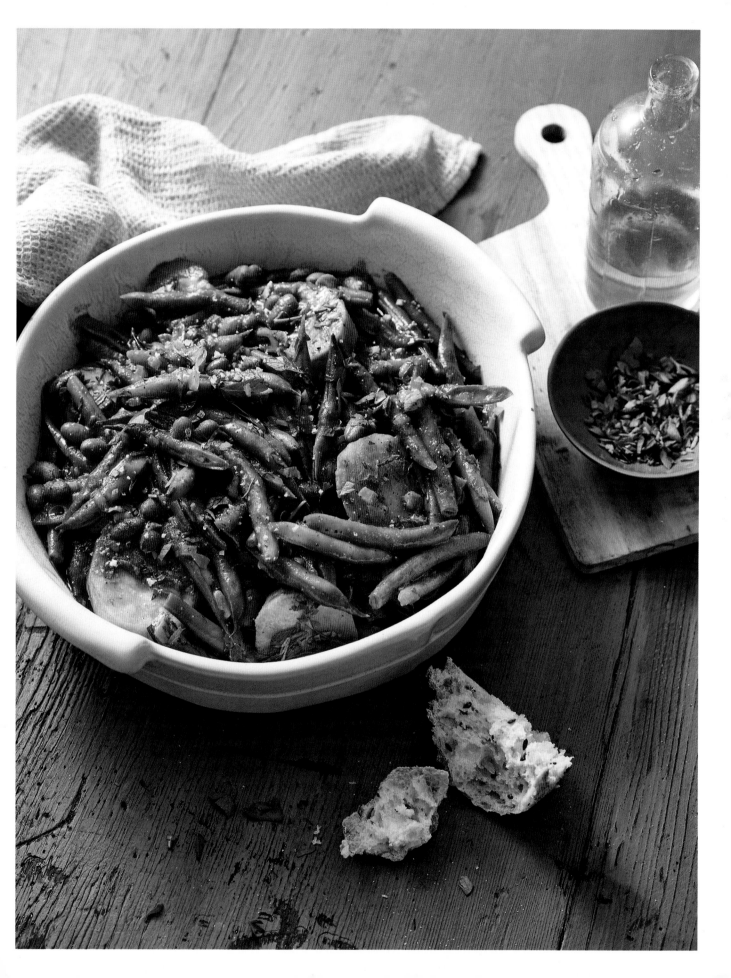

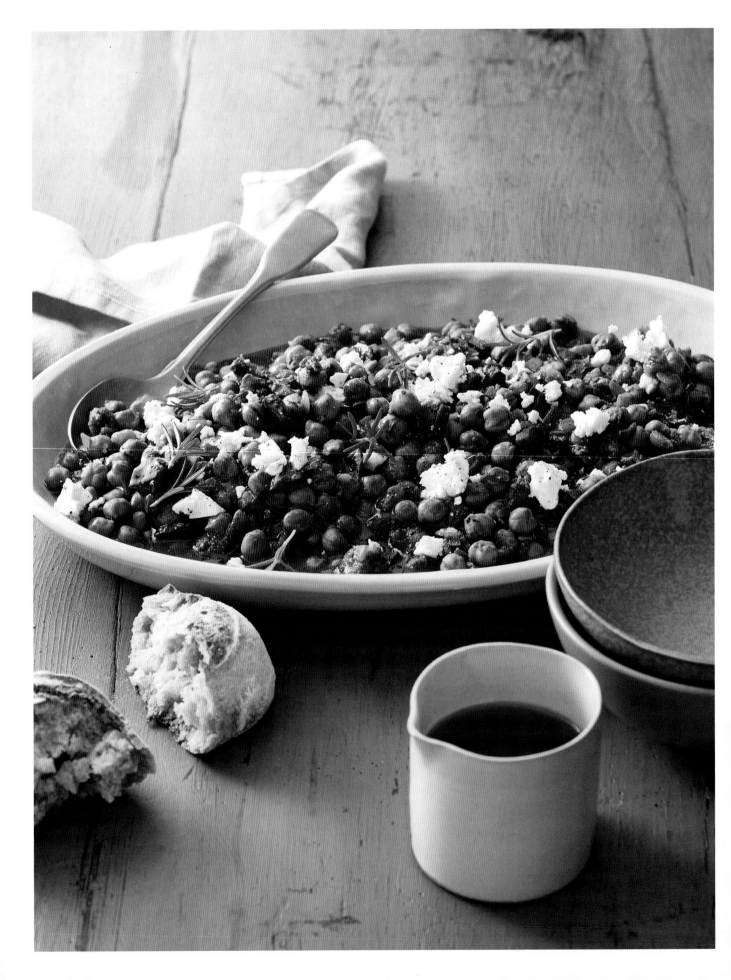

Chickpea and rosemary casserole

Extra-virgin olive oil

1 red onion, finely diced

1 small red chilli, halved, deseeded and finely chopped or pinch chilli flakes

2 garlic cloves, finely diced

1 red capsicum, deseeded and diced

3 x 400 g tins chickpeas, drained and rinsed

½ cup (125 ml) red wine

2–3 rosemary sprigs, leaves picked and chopped, plus extra to serve

½ teaspoon ground cinnamon

1 x 400 g tin crushed tomatoes

2 cups (500 ml) boiling water

Sea salt and freshly ground black pepper

30 g feta, crumbled

This dish was inspired during a recent trip to the Greek island of Zakynthos. The fresh rosemary and cinnamon add amazing flavours to the chickpeas, especially when topped with a little feta.

Heat the olive oil in a large heavy-based saucepan over a medium heat and sauté the onion and chilli until the onion is softened and translucent. Add the garlic, capsicum, chickpeas and red wine and simmer until the alcohol has mostly evaporated.

Add the rosemary and cinnamon to the pan and stir through. Add the tomatoes and boiling water, then simmer for 10–15 minutes, or until the mixture thickens. Season with salt and pepper to taste.

Serve, topped with the extra rosemary and crumbled feta.

Nutrient	Average Qty per serving	%RDI F	M
NUTRITION COMPOSITION PER SERVE			
Energy	1684 kj	20%	16%
Protein	16.1 g	22%	18%
Carbohydrate	31.4 g	13%	10%
Fat	18.1 g	23%	18%
Sodium	730 mg	37%	37%
Fibre	16.4 g	59%	43%

High in fibre and calcium

Stuffed *baby pumpkins* with pumpkin and turmeric yoghurt

COOKING

1

HOUR +
30 MINUTES

SERVES

6

STUFFED BABY PUMPKINS

6 baby butternut pumpkins

½ cup (70 g) mixed seeds

1 cup (200 g) rice (jasmine, basmati, or wild rice)

1 tablespoon extra-virgin olive oil, plus extra for drizzling

1 cup (250 ml) vegetable stock

1 cup (250 ml) water

¼ teaspoon ground nutmeg

Sea salt and freshly ground black pepper

PUMPKIN AND TURMERIC YOGHURT

200 g pumpkin (any type), peeled and diced (use scooped out flesh from the prepared baby butternut pumpkins)

⅓ cup (90 g) thick Greek-style yoghurt

½ teaspoon ground turmeric

¼ teaspoon smoked paprika

TO SERVE

Fresh herbs, if on hand

Leafy green salad

This impressive looking dish is a variation on the traditional stuffed capsicums, with great contrast of flavours from the sweet pumpkin and the spicy turmeric-flavoured yoghurt dressing.

Preheat the oven to 200°C. Use a sharp knife to cut the top off each baby pumpkin. Set aside the tops. Cut another 3 cm piece off the top of each pumpkin to make them smaller. Remove the seeds and some of the pumpkin flesh to create a cavity for stuffing. Peel and dice the 3 cm pieces and the scooped out pumpkin flesh.

Place the diced pumpkin for the pumpkin and turmeric yoghurt on a roasting tray, drizzle with the olive oil and roast for 30 minutes. Remove and set aside to cool. Turn the oven down to 180°C.

Heat a large heavy-based frying pan over a medium–low heat and gently toast the mixed seeds until golden, taking care not to burn them, then transfer to a plate. Return the pan to the heat, add the rice and 1 tablespoon of olive oil to the frying pan, and sauté until the rice is well coated in oil.

Return the toasted seeds to the pan. Add the vegetable stock and water and simmer for 15 minutes to par-cook the rice. Add the nutmeg and season with salt and pepper. Remove the pan from the heat and cool the rice mixture. Divide the cooled rice mixture between the baby pumpkins, filling each one nearly to the top.

Arrange the stuffed pumpkins on a baking tray, pop their lids back on and bake for 45 minutes–1 hour, or until the pumpkins and rice are cooked.

Put the roasted pumpkin for the yoghurt into a food processor, add the yoghurt, turmeric and smoked paprika and blend until smooth. Taste, then season with salt and pepper and adjust the flavours, if needed.

Garnish the stuffed pumpkins with the fresh herbs, if on hand, add a generous drizzle of pumpkin and turmeric yoghurt and serve with a leafy green salad.

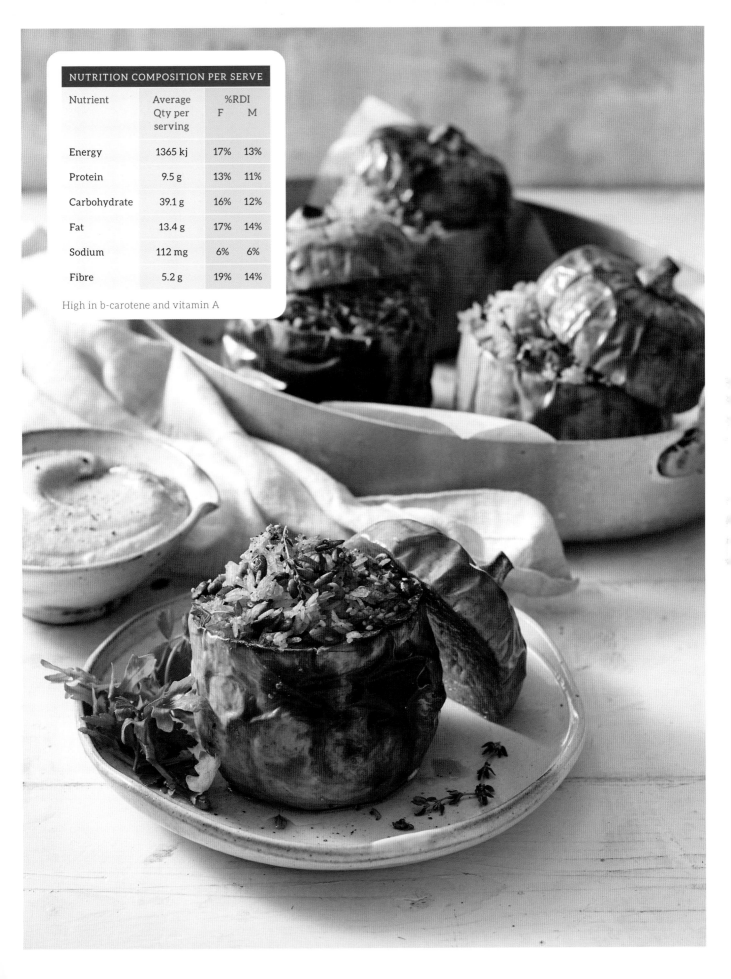

NUTRITION COMPOSITION PER SERVE

Nutrient	Average Qty per serving	%RDI F	M
Energy	1365 kj	17%	13%
Protein	9.5 g	13%	11%
Carbohydrate	39.1 g	16%	12%
Fat	13.4 g	17%	14%
Sodium	112 mg	6%	6%
Fibre	5.2 g	19%	14%

High in b-carotene and vitamin A

Cauliflower steaks
with turmeric yoghurt

COOKING
30
MINUTES

SERVES
4
AS A SIDE

1 head of purple or white cauliflower

Extra-virgin olive oil

Sea salt and freshly ground black pepper

Smoked paprika, plus extra to serve

TURMERIC YOGHURT

1 cup (250 g) thick Greek-style yoghurt

2 tablespoons tahini

1 teaspoon ground turmeric

¼ teaspoon smoked paprika

1 teaspoon lemon juice

2 teaspoons roughly chopped preserved
  lemon rind (see page 207)

TO SERVE

Fresh herbs, if on hand

Small red chilli, finely chopped or sliced

Optional: crushed pistachios

This dish is not just for vegetarians. The cauliflower steaks are combined with aromatic spices and pistachios to boost the anti-inflammatory nutrients.

Preheat the oven to 180°C. Line a large baking tray with baking paper.

Carefully slice 1 cm thick slices of cauliflower from the top to the base to make four 'steaks'. Arrange flat on the baking tray, drizzle with the olive oil and season with salt and pepper and a few pinches of smoked paprika. Bake for 20–30 minutes, then set aside to cool.

Prepare the turmeric yoghurt by combining the yoghurt, tahini, turmeric, smoked paprika, lemon juice and preserved lemon in a small bowl. Season with salt and pepper to taste, then set aside.

Arrange the cauliflower steaks on a platter or on individual plates, then drizzle 1 or 2 tablespoons of turmeric yoghurt over the top. Garnish with the fresh herbs, if on hand, some chilli and pistachios (if using), then sprinkle over a little smoked paprika and serve.

NUTRITION COMPOSITION PER SERVE			
Nutrient	Average Qty per serving	%RDI F	M
Energy	1115 kj	14%	11%
Protein	7.6 g	10%	8%
Carbohydrate	8 g	3%	3%
Fat	22 g	28%	22%
Sodium	162 mg	8%	8%
Fibre	3.4 g	12%	9%

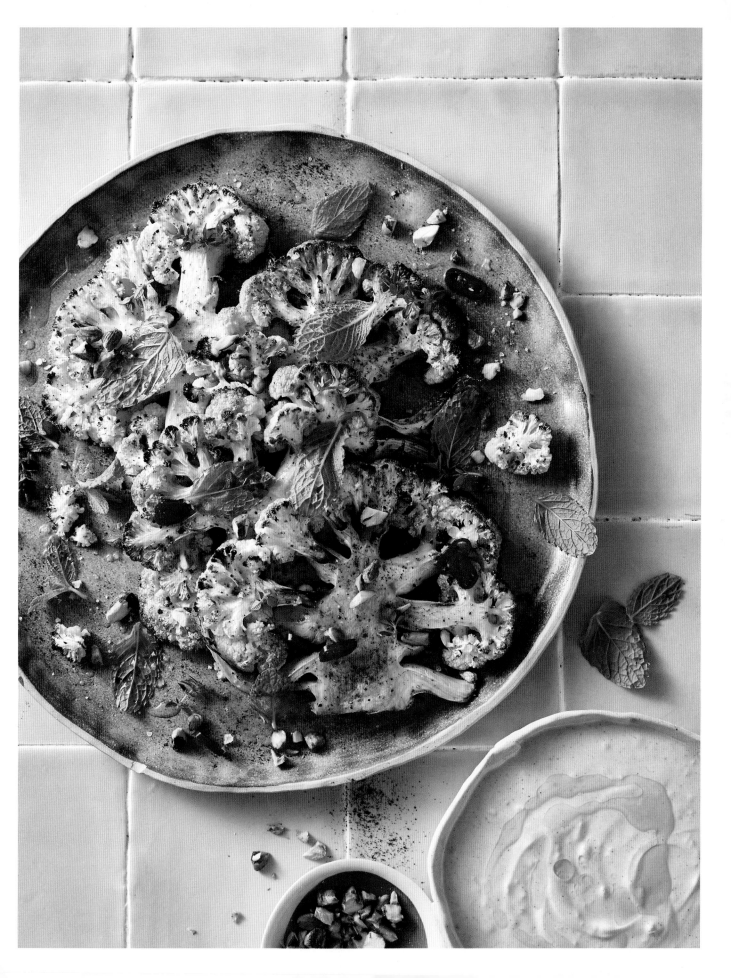

Village-style *sourdough* bride

COOKING	MAKES
50 MINUTES	**1** LOAF

200 g sourdough starter
   (see recipe below)

2½ cups (375 ml) lukewarm water

1 teaspoon fine salt (iodised, if possible)

1 tablespoon honey

200 g wholemeal flour, sifted

100 g maize flour, sifted

100 g rye flour, sifted

600 g white bread flour, sifted

¼ cup (60 ml) extra-virgin olive oil,
   plus extra for greasing

2 tablespoons sesame seeds

SOURDOUGH STARTER (PROZIMI) (SEE NOTE)

½ cup (125 ml) lukewarm water

60 g fresh yeast

½ cup (100 g) bread flour

Step 1: Make the sourdough starter. Put the warm water in a bowl, then crumble the yeast into it and add the flour. Mix well, cover and allow to stand overnight in a warm spot in the house. The yeast will develop and become sour and foamy, giving the bread a characteristic flavour and texture.

If making by hand

Step 2: Lightly oil a large mixing bowl, then set aside.

Step 3: In a large mixing bowl use a wooden spoon to mix the sourdough starter with the water, salt, honey and wholemeal, maize and rye flour until well combined.

Step 4: Slowly add the white bread flour and knead the mixture with lightly oiled hands until a soft dough forms.

Step 5: Place the dough in the oiled bowl and cover with a cloth. Place in a warm spot and allow to rise for about an hour, or until doubled in size.

If using a bread maker

Step 2: Make sure the machine is on the 'dough' setting.

Step 3: Add the yeast mixture to a 1 kg loaf bowl. Slowly add the sifted flours while the mixing element is on.

Step 4: Add the salt, honey and 300 ml of warm water.

Step 5: Allow the flour mixture to knead in the bread maker and then rise.

Step 1 of cooking: Preheat the oven to 180°C. Generously oil a loaf tin, then line with baking paper.

Step 2 of cooking: Transfer the dough mixture to the lined tin, then sprinkle with the sesame seeds.

Step 3 of cooking: Bake for 45–50 minutes, or until the loaf is golden brown and sounds hollow when tapped. Cool in the tin for 10 minutes, then turn out onto a wire rack and slice as needed.

NOTE

As an alternative to making your own sourdough starter, you can use 2 tablespoons of dried yeast (2 packets). Place the dried yeast in a large bowl and add 2½ cups (625 ml) of lukewarm water and fine salt, stir and allow to stand for 10 minutes.

NUTRITION COMPOSITION PER SERVE*

Nutrient	Average Qty per serving	%RDI F	M
Energy	1085 kj	13%	11%
Protein	7.2 g	10%	8%
Carbohydrate	44.3 g	18%	14%
Fat	4.9 g	6%	5%
Sodium	208 mg	10%	10%
Fibre	3.6 g	13%	9%

*2 slices (90 g) sourdough bread per serve

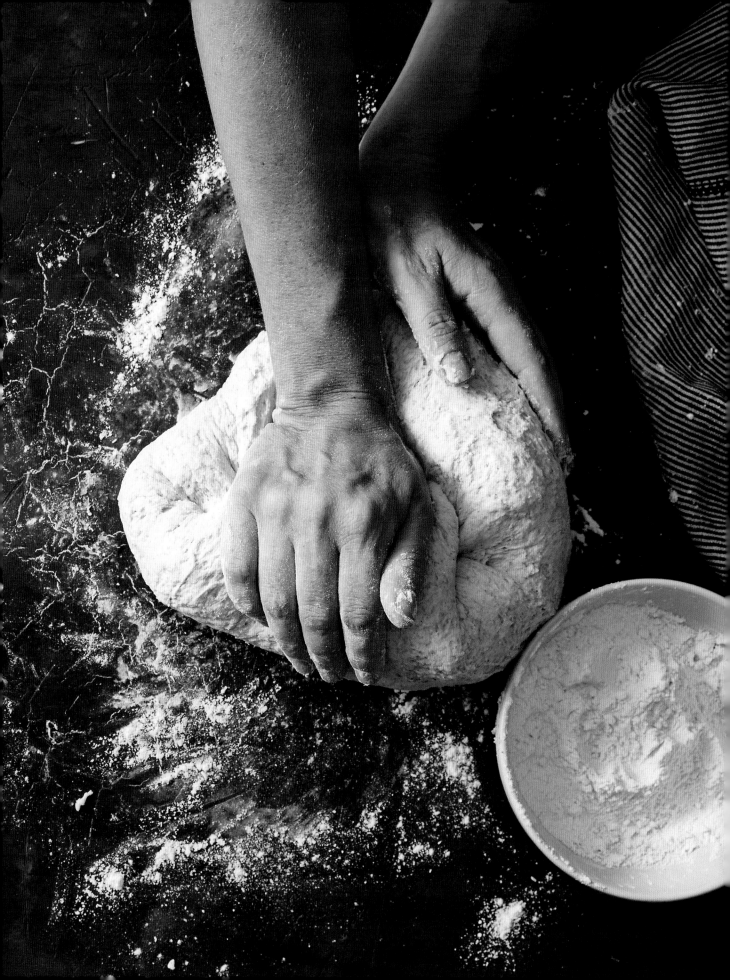

Lahanodolmades:
vegetarian cabbage rolls

COOKING
1
HOUR +
20 MINUTES

SERVES
6
MAKES 12
ROLLS

1 cabbage (purple, if possible)

Boiling water

60–80 ml (¼–⅓ cup) extra-virgin olive oil,
plus extra for drizzling

1 small red onion, finely diced

Optional: ½ teaspoon chopped small red
chilli or chilli flakes

1 small purple sweet potato, peeled and
finely diced (or grated)

2 tablespoons chopped dill

2 tablespoons chopped flat-leaf parsley

60 g pine nuts

2 tablespoons currants

1 cup (200 g) rice (jasmine, basmati
or brown)

½ teaspoon ground nutmeg

Sea salt and freshly ground black pepper

4 tomatoes, skinned, grated and puréed
(see tip on page 97)

Salad or sautéed wild greens, to serve

EGG AND LEMON SAUCE

2 eggs

Juice 1 lemon

I have varied the classic Greek cabbage rolls with egg and lemon sauce from my first book to make this vegetarian version with pine nuts, currants and aromatic spices. My husband calls them 'Greek dim sims' and they were his favourite dish from his mother-in-law. He thinks these are okay too. He is eating more vegetarian these days.

Prepare the cabbage leaves first. Trim the stem at the base so the leaves separate easily when cooked. Place in a large saucepan, cover with boiling water and simmer for 30 minutes, or until the leaves are soft. Drain and allow to cool before separating the leaves (you'll need about 8–10 large leaves for this).

Heat the olive oil in a heavy-based saucepan over a medium heat and sauté the onion and chilli (if using) for 3–4 minutes, or until the onion is translucent. Add the sweet potato, dill, parsley, pine nuts, currants and rice, then season with the nutmeg, salt and pepper to taste, and stir well. Add ½ cup (125 ml) of the puréed tomato and 5 cups (1.25 litres) of boiling water and simmer for 10–15 minutes, or until the rice is almost cooked, then set aside to cool.

Place a cabbage leaf on a board and put 2–3 tablespoons of the rice mixture at the base of the leaf. Fold in the sides, then roll up towards the top to make a parcel. Repeat until the rest of the cabbage leaves and filling have been used.

Place the cabbage rolls, seam side down, in a large pot with a lid, packing them in tightly together. Pour 4 cups (1 litre) of boiling water slowly over the cabbage rolls until they are almost covered, then drizzle a little olive oil over the top. Place a heatproof plate on top of the rolls to keep them from opening while they cook. Put the lid on the pot, then place over a medium heat and simmer for 30 minutes. Once cooked, set aside to cool and remove the plate.

Prepare the egg and lemon sauce by beating the eggs together and gradually beating in the lemon juice. Slowly pour this sauce over the cabbage rolls and swirl the pot around to ensure they are well covered.

Serve hot with a lettuce and cucumber salad or Sautéed wild greens (see page 89).

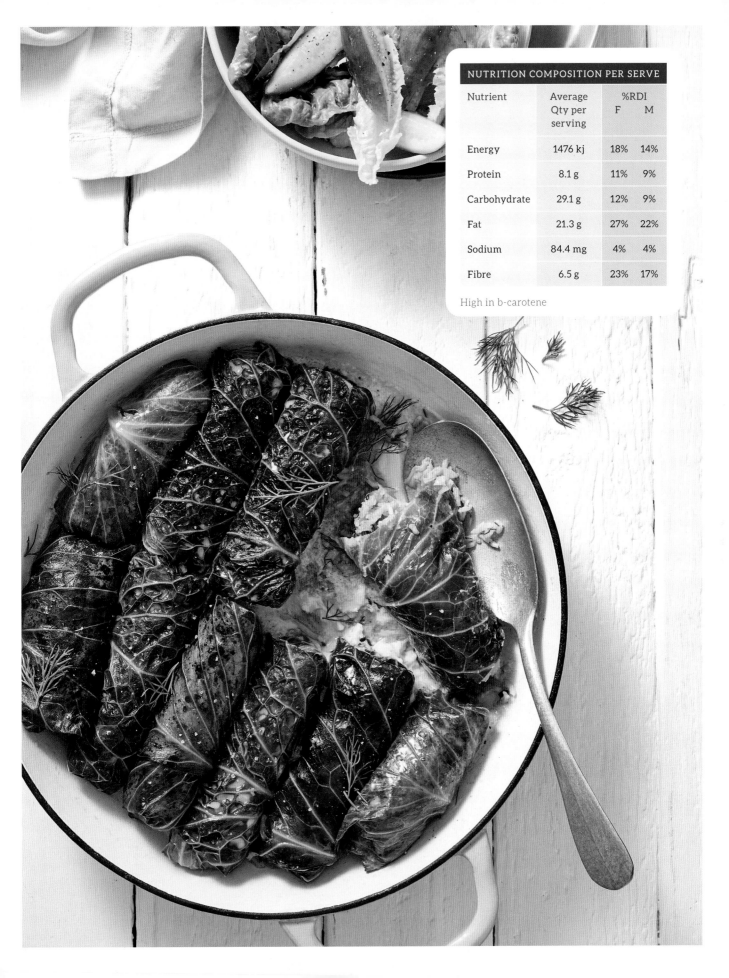

NUTRITION COMPOSITION PER SERVE

Nutrient	Average Qty per serving	%RDI F	M
Energy	1476 kj	18%	14%
Protein	8.1 g	11%	9%
Carbohydrate	29.1 g	12%	9%
Fat	21.3 g	27%	22%
Sodium	84.4 mg	4%	4%
Fibre	6.5 g	23%	17%

High in b-carotene

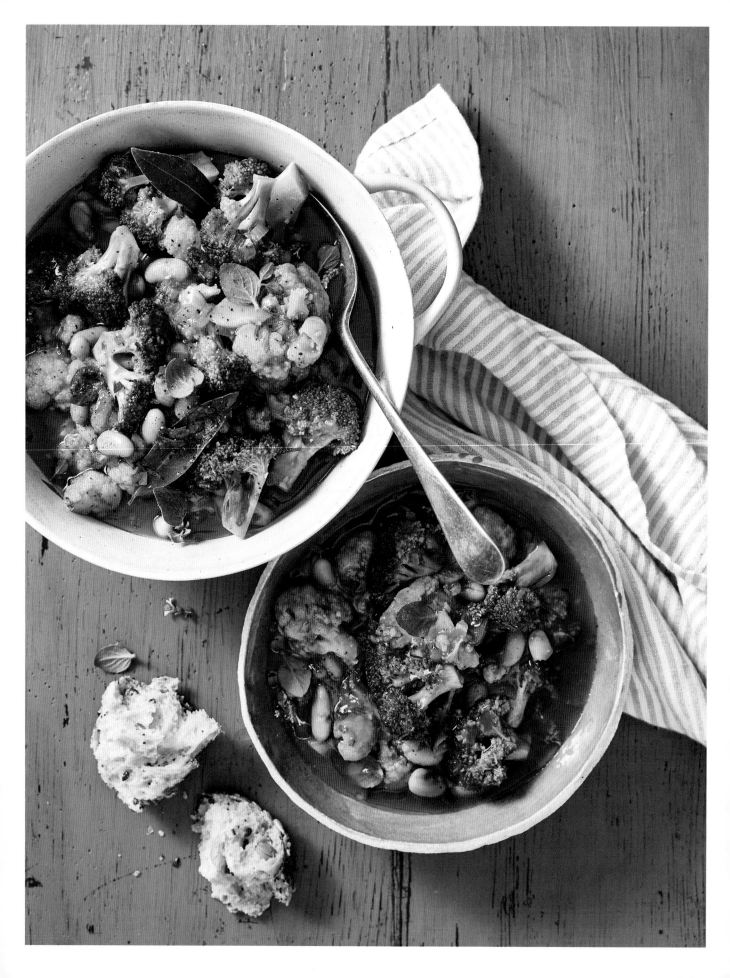

Cauliflower and broccoli
with cannellini beans

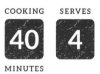

COOKING 40 MINUTES

SERVES 4

¼ cup (60 ml) olive oil

1 red onion, finely chopped

1 small red chilli, halved, deseeded
and finely sliced

300 g cauliflower, cut into florets

300 g broccoli, cut into florets

1 cup (250 ml) puréed tomato

3–4 fresh bay leaves

2–3 flat-leaf parsley sprigs,
finely chopped

2 garlic cloves, crushed

Sea salt and freshly ground black pepper

1 x 400 g tin cannellini beans, drained
and rinsed

2 cups (500 ml) boiling water, as needed

Dried oregano

Fresh herbs, if on hand

Seasonal vegetables cooked in a rich tomato sauce with onion, garlic, herbs and extra-virgin olive oil are often called yiahni-style in Greek. This dish swaps out the common green beans for cruciferous vegetables and legumes to boost protein and fibre.

Heat the olive oil in a large heavy-based saucepan over a medium heat and sauté the onion and chilli for 1–2 minutes, or until they start to soften.

Add the cauliflower and broccoli florets to the pan and sauté for 5 minutes. Add the tomato, bay leaves, parsley and garlic, then season with salt and pepper to taste. Add the cannellini beans and stir well.

Pour in enough boiling water to cover the vegetables and simmer for 30 minutes, or until the vegetables are cooked through.

Taste, and add the oregano to your liking. Adjust the seasonings if necessary and serve with the fresh herbs, if on hand.

TIP

Pair this dish with the sourdough bread (see page 106) to mop up the sauce, or a leafy green salad for a lower kilojoule option.

NUTRITION COMPOSITION PER SERVE			
Nutrient	Average Qty per serving	%RDI F	M
Energy	1106 kj	13%	11%
Protein	10.4 g	14%	12%
Carbohydrate	14.8 g	6%	5%
Fat	15.9 g	20%	16%
Sodium	417 mg	21%	21%
Fibre	10.2 g	36%	27%

High in vitamin C and folate
and good source of fibre

Beetroot, tahini and yoghurt dip

1 large or 2 small beetroots (see intro)

⅓ cup (90 g) thick Greek-style yoghurt

1 tablespoon tahini

1 tablespoon extra-virgin olive oil, plus extra for drizzling

¼ preserved lemon rind (see page 207), finely diced

¼ teaspoon ground cumin

Sea salt and freshly ground black pepper

Optional: sourdough toast (see page 106), to serve

I love this bright, tasty dip because it has multiple uses: I serve it as part of a mezze platter with crusty bread, crackers or veggie sticks, use it instead of butter as a spread on burgers or sandwiches or where I'd use another creamy sauce. If you are short on time, you can use the pre-cooked beetroot available from supermarkets and skip the roasting.

Preheat the oven to 200°C. Line a baking tray with baking paper and wrap the beetroot(s) in foil. Roast for 30–45 minutes, or until a knife passes easily through the beetroot, then remove from the oven and allow to cool.

Blend the roasted beetroot in a food processor until creamy, then transfer to a bowl and mix in the yoghurt and tahini until well combined. Add the olive oil, preserved lemon and cumin. Season with salt and pepper to taste, then serve right away with a drizzle of olive oil and the sourdough toast (if using) or store until needed. This dip can be kept in an airtight container in the fridge for up to 5 days.

NUTRITION COMPOSITION PER SERVE*		%RDI	
Nutrient	Average Qty per serving	F	M
Energy	754 kj	9%	7%
Protein	2.5 g	3%	3%
Carbohydrate	4.8 g	2%	2%
Fat	9.2 g	12%	9%
Sodium	66 mg	3%	3%
Fibre	1.5 g	5%	4%

*Dip only

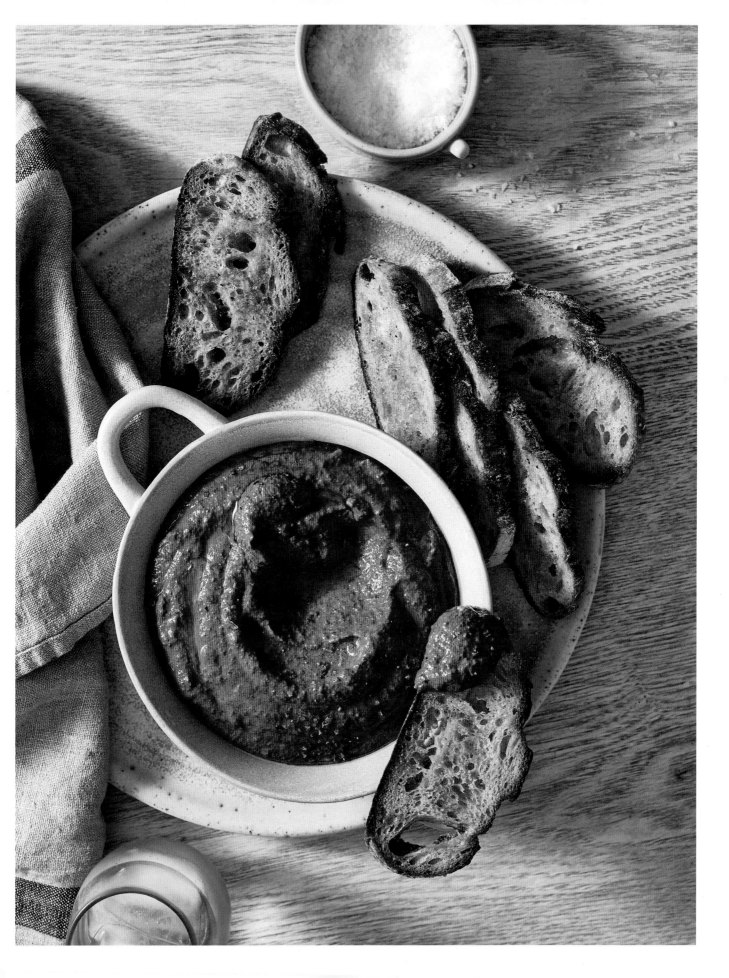

Mushroom and asparagus frittata

2 tablespoons extra-virgin olive oil

1 red onion, finely chopped

2¼ cups (200 g) cleaned and sliced button mushrooms

1 bunch (100 g) asparagus, cut into 2 cm pieces

1 small red chilli, finely sliced

1 tablespoon picked thyme leaves

½ bunch (100 g) spring onions, chopped

5 eggs, lightly beaten

Sea salt and freshly ground black pepper

Fresh herbs, if on hand

Here is a tasty way to enjoy a quick vegetarian meal when asparagus is in season. My family enjoy chilli so I add it to everything, especially eggs.

Heat the olive oil in a large heavy-based frying pan over a medium heat and sauté the red onion until softened and translucent. Add the mushroom and sauté for 5 minutes.

Add the asparagus, chilli, thyme and spring onion to the pan, and sauté for 5 minutes.

Gently pour the lightly beaten egg over the top of the mushroom mixture and swirl around the frying pan to ensure the egg is well distributed over the sautéed vegetables. Cook for a few minutes, until the egg has set.

Season the frittata with salt and pepper, then garnish with the fresh herbs, if on hand, before serving.

NUTRITION COMPOSITION PER SERVE			
Nutrient	Average Qty per serving	%RDI F	M
Energy	859 kj	10%	8%
Protein	11.1 g	15%	12%
Carbohydrate	4.2 g	2%	1%
Fat	15.1 g	19%	15%
Sodium	186 mg	9%	9%
Fibre	3.8 g	14%	10%

Mushroom and orzo 'risotto'

2 tablespoons extra-virgin olive oil,
 plus extra for frying

300 g Swiss brown mushrooms, cleaned
 and sliced

1 onion, finely chopped

500 g orzo pasta

1 cup (250 ml) dry white wine

40 g dried porcini mushrooms, soaked
 in 1 cup (250 ml) boiling water for
 10 minutes

4 cups (1 litre) hot vegetable stock

50 g butter or dairy-free margarine

½ cup (50 g) grated parmesan cheese

Sea salt and freshly ground black pepper

Fresh herbs, if on hand

Orzo or risoni is a fine pasta that resembles long-grain rice. It is commonly used in Greek cuisine in baked pasta dishes but works beautifully in this rich mushroom risotto.

Heat a drizzle of olive oil in a large frying pan over a medium heat, then sauté the mushroom for 10 minutes and set aside.

Heat 2 tablespoons of olive oil in a large heavy-based saucepan over a medium heat and sauté the onion until softened and translucent. Add the orzo and continue to cook, stirring, until the orzo is coated in the oil and starts to turn white (don't let it burn). Add the wine, and stir over the heat until most of the alcohol cooks off.

Remove the soaked porcini mushrooms from the water (reserve their soaking water) and finely slice them. Add to the orzo mixture along with their soaking water.

Gradually stir in half of the hot vegetable stock (about a cup at a time) – wait for each cup to absorb before adding the next. Once the stock has been added, stir through the sautéed mushrooms. Continue gradually adding the rest of the vegetable stock until the orzo is cooked (it should have a fairly moist consistency – not dry and not too soupy). You may need to add some boiling water if the orzo needs more cooking.

Once the orzo is cooked, stir through the butter or margarine and parmesan cheese, season with salt and pepper to taste and garnish with the fresh herbs, if on hand, to serve.

TIP

If you prefer vegan and don't want to use vegan dairy substitutes, the dish can be finished with an extra drizzle of extra-virgin olive oil and a tablespoon of crushed walnuts or hazelnuts.

NUTRITION COMPOSITION PER SERVE			
Nutrient	Average Qty per serving	%RDI F	M
Energy	2006 kj	24%	20%
Protein	16.1 g	22%	18%
Carbohydrate	59.1 g	24%	18%
Fat	17.4 g	22%	18%
Sodium	682 mg	34%	34%
Fibre	4 g	14%	11%

Lentil pilaf

COOKING **40** MINUTES

SERVES **6** AS A SIDE

2 tablespoons extra-virgin olive oil

1 small onion, finely chopped

2 cups (400 g) basmati rice

¼ teaspoon ground cumin

¼ teaspoon saffron threads

¼ teaspoon ground allspice

3–4 cloves

1 x 400 g tin brown lentils, drained
   and rinsed

5 cups (1.25 litres) hot vegetable stock

3 tablespoons currants

3 tablespoons crushed pistachios

Sea salt and freshly ground black pepper

Baby kale, fresh herbs and lemon wedges,
   if on hand

This dish is a variation of the classic Cypriot rice and lentil pilaf (fakes moutzentra) with added aromatic spices, currants and fresh herbs for flavour and a boost of antioxidants. It is also common in the Middle East where the dish is known as mujaddara and is topped with fried onions.

Heat the olive oil in a large heavy-based saucepan over a medium heat and sauté the onion until softened and translucent. Add the rice and cook, stirring, for 5 minutes, making sure the grains are well coated in the oil. Add the spices and continue to cook for a few more minutes. Add the lentils and vegetable stock, stir well and simmer with the lid on until most of the liquid has been absorbed.

Remove the pan from the heat and cover with a clean tea towel, then place the lid tightly on top. Allow to sit for 15 minutes – this allows the extra liquid to evaporate and makes the rice fluffy.

When ready, stir through the currants and pistachios, season with salt and pepper to taste and garnish with the kale, fresh herbs and lemon wedges, if on hand.

NUTRITION COMPOSITION PER SERVE			
Nutrient	Average Qty per serving	%RDI F	M
Energy	1657 kj	20%	16%
Protein	10.6 g	15%	12%
Carbohydrate	63.6 g	25%	20%
Fat	9.7 g	12%	10%
Sodium	90 mg	5%	5%
Fibre	4.2 g	15%	11%

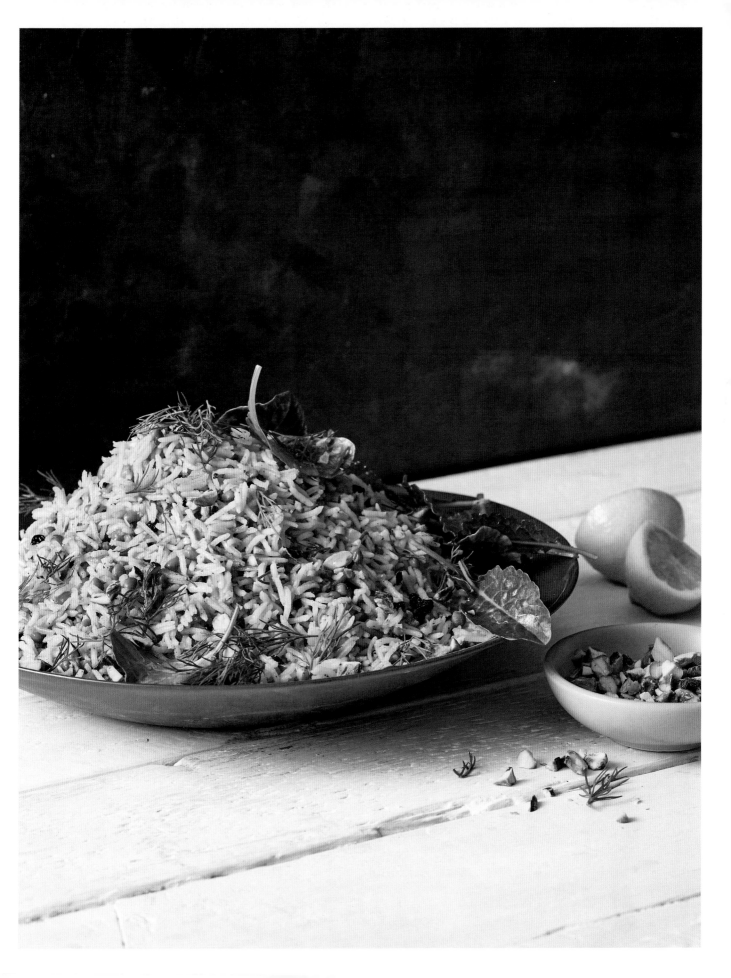

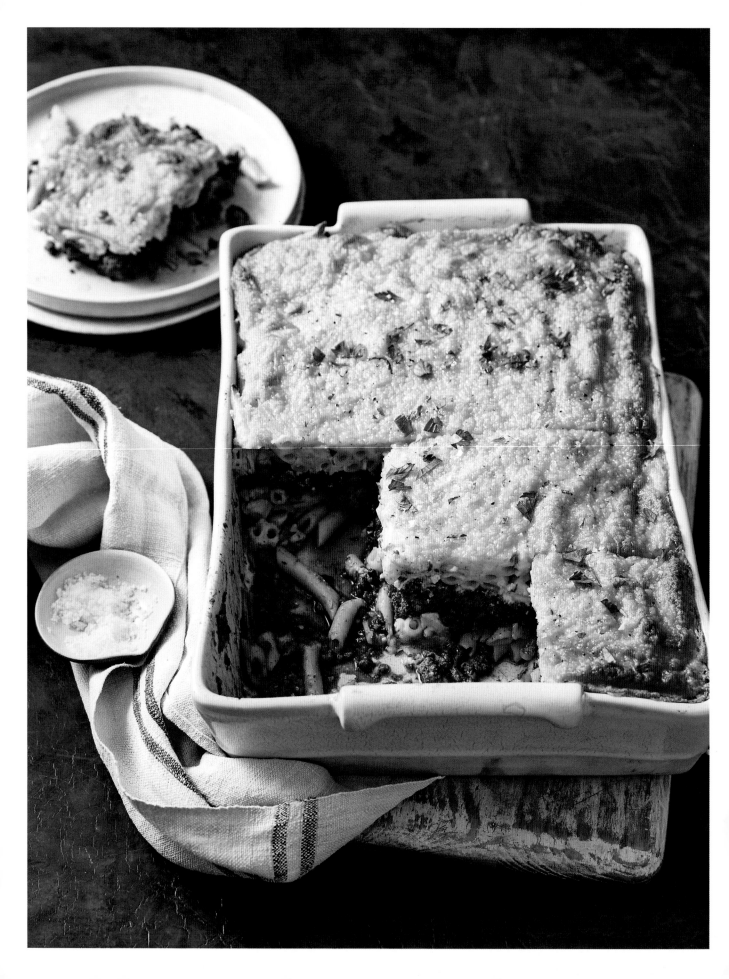

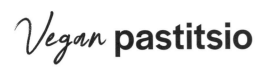 **pastitsio**

½ cup (125 ml) extra-virgin olive oil

1 onion, finely chopped

2 garlic cloves, finely diced

100 g flat mushrooms, finely diced

1 eggplant, finely diced

500 g vegan mince, such as Quorn

½ cup (125 ml) red wine

1 x 400 g tin chopped tomatoes

1 cup (250 ml) puréed tomato

Sea salt and freshly ground black pepper

1 small red chilli, halved, deseeded
   and finely chopped or ½ teaspoon
   chilli flakes

½ teaspoon mixed dried herbs

500 g penne pasta

150 g vegan feta

2 tablespoons finely chopped flat-leaf
   parsley, plus extra to serve

Leafy green salad, to serve

BECHAMEL

100 g dairy-free margarine

100 g plain flour

2 cups (500 ml) soy milk or other vegan
   alternative such as oat or almond milk

My daughter Vivienne and I designed this vegan version of a traditional pastitsio, which normally has a meat sauce, for a party with friends who were strictly vegan. Our non-vegetarian friends were also impressed.

Heat the olive oil in a large frying pan and sauté the onion until softened and translucent. Add the garlic, mushrooms and eggplant and sauté for 10 minutes. Add the vegan mince and red wine and simmer until the alcohol has evaporated.

Add the tinned and puréed tomatoes and 500 ml water. Season with salt and pepper to taste and then add the chilli and mixed dried herbs and simmer for 15–20 minutes.

Meanwhile, cook the pasta in salted boiling water with a few drops of olive oil until al dente. Once cooked, drain and then splash a little olive oil on the pasta.

To make the bechamel, melt the margarine in a heavy-based saucepan over a medium–low heat, then add the flour to make a roux. Slowly add the soy milk until creamy, whisking as you go. If lumps form, whisk vigorously until they disappear.

To assemble the pastitsio, layer half of the pasta around the base of a large baking dish. Spoon a thick layer of the vegan mince sauce on top, then crumble over the vegan feta. Cover with the remaining pasta, then spoon and spread the bechamel evenly over the top. Bake in the oven for 45–50 minutes, or until golden brown on top.

Allow the pastitsio to cool slightly for 10–15 minutes, then cut into 4 cm square portions, scatter over the parsley and serve with a leafy green salad.

NUTRITION COMPOSITION PER SERVE			
Nutrient	Average Qty per serving	%RDI F	M
Energy	2669 kj	32%	26%
Protein	18 g	25%	20%
Carbohydrate	65.6 g	26%	21%
Fat	31.7 g	40%	32%
Sodium	510 mg	26%	26%
Fibre	7.5 g	27%	20%

Seasonal *vegetable bake* with goat's feta

COOKING **55** MINUTES

SERVES **4**

2 red onions, quartered

200 g baby zucchini, halved lengthways

200 g baby eggplants, halved lengthways

100 g long green chillies, deseeded
and cut into 2 cm pieces

100 g green capsicum, deseeded
and cut into 2 cm pieces

1 small red chilli, halved, deseeded
and finely sliced

¼ cup (60 ml) extra-virgin olive oil

2 tomatoes, grated (see tip on page 97)

200 g cherry tomatoes, halved if large

2 cups (500 ml) boiling water

1 tablespoon oregano leaves

Sea salt and freshly ground black pepper

50 g goat's feta, crumbled

Fresh herbs, if on hand

On a recent trip to the Greek island of Zakynthos my husband, Savvas, and I rented a house. Our welcome basket included eggs and local extra-virgin olive oil as well as fresh vegetables from the garden: zucchini, eggplants, capsicums, onions, cherry tomatoes and herbs. I was inspired to whip up this seasonal vegetable bake and it tasted delicious!

This dish can be baked in the oven or prepared in a casserole dish with a lid and cooked on the stovetop. Baking the vegetables for a longer time allows them to caramelise and produce a richer flavour.

If you plan on baking this dish rather than cooking on the stovetop, preheat the oven to 180°C.

Place the onion, zucchini, eggplant, green chilli, capsicum and red chilli in a large flameproof casserole or baking dish over a medium heat and add the olive oil. Sauté for 10 minutes, or until the vegetables start to soften.

Add the grated tomato and cherry tomatoes along with the boiling water to the dish. Season with the oregano and salt and pepper, then cook over a low heat for 30 minutes, or bake for 45 minutes.

Before serving, crumble the feta over the baked vegetables and garnish with the fresh herbs, if on hand.

NUTRITION COMPOSITION PER SERVE			
Nutrient	Average Qty per serving	%RDI F	M
Energy	1004 kj	12%	10%
Protein	6.2 g	8%	7%
Carbohydrate	11.5 g	5%	4%
Fat	17.2 g	22%	18%
Sodium	239 mg	12%	12%
Fibre	8 g	29%	21%

High in vitamin C and b-carotene
and good source of fibre

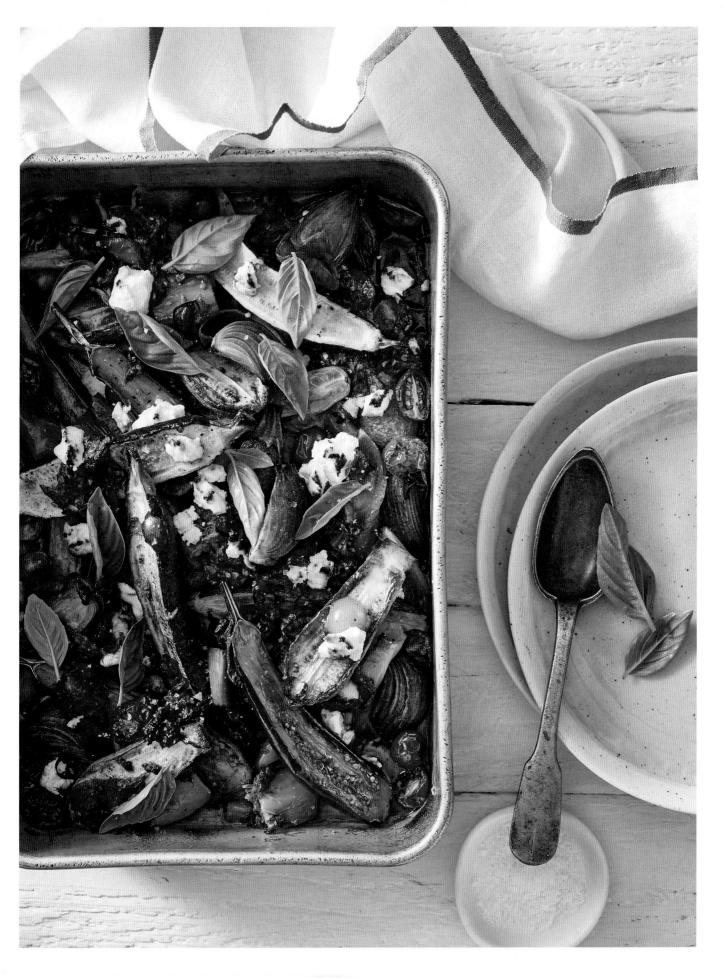

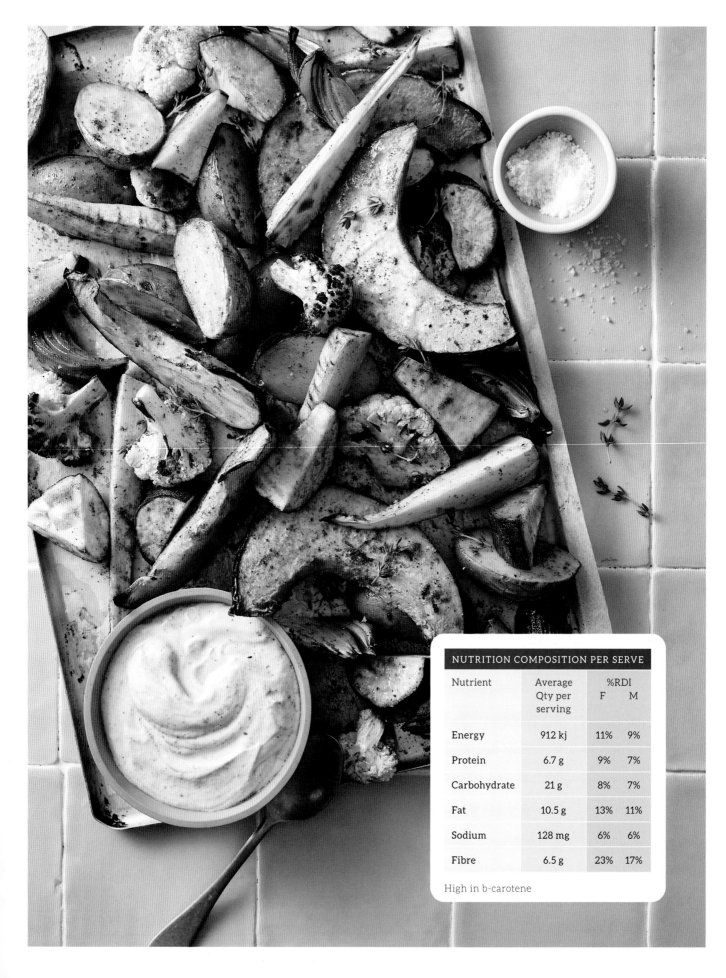

NUTRITION COMPOSITION PER SERVE

Nutrient	Average Qty per serving	%RDI F	%RDI M
Energy	912 kj	11%	9%
Protein	6.7 g	9%	7%
Carbohydrate	21 g	8%	7%
Fat	10.5 g	13%	11%
Sodium	128 mg	6%	6%
Fibre	6.5 g	23%	17%

High in b-carotene

Roasted vegetables with spiced tahini yoghurt

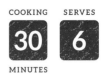

200 g cauliflower, cut into florets

300 g Kent pumpkin, skin on, cut into
  2 cm wedges

4 small red onions, quartered

200 g purple or orange sweet potato,
  skin on, cut into 2 cm pieces

200 g baby royal blue potatoes,
  skin on, halved

200 g parsnip, skin on, cut into
  2 cm pieces

2 tablespoons extra-virgin olive oil

½ teaspoon smoked paprika, plus extra
  to serve

½ teaspoon ground cumin

¼ teaspoon mustard powder

Sea salt and freshly ground black pepper

Fresh herbs, if on hand

SPICED TAHINI YOGHURT

½ cup (120 g) thick Greek-style yoghurt

1 tablespoon tahini

¼ teaspoon ground cumin

¼ teaspoon mustard powder

¼ teaspoon smoked paprika

A quick and healthy way to enjoy any leftover vegetables. Mixing starchy and non-starchy vegetables – dressed with extra-virgin olive oil, aromatic spices and yoghurt – makes this dish a substantial vegetarian option.

Preheat the oven to 180°C. Put all the vegetables into a large roasting tin or divide between two tins, if necessary. Drizzle over the olive oil and add the paprika, cumin and mustard powder and season with salt and pepper to taste. Use your hands to toss the vegetables and coat them in the flavours.

Add ½ cup (125 ml) of water to the roasting tin, then bake for 30 minutes, or until the root vegetables are cooked through.

Prepare the spiced tahini yoghurt by mixing all the ingredients well in a bowl. Drizzle this mixture all over the vegetables, then garnish with the fresh herbs, if on hand, and a sprinkle of extra paprika.

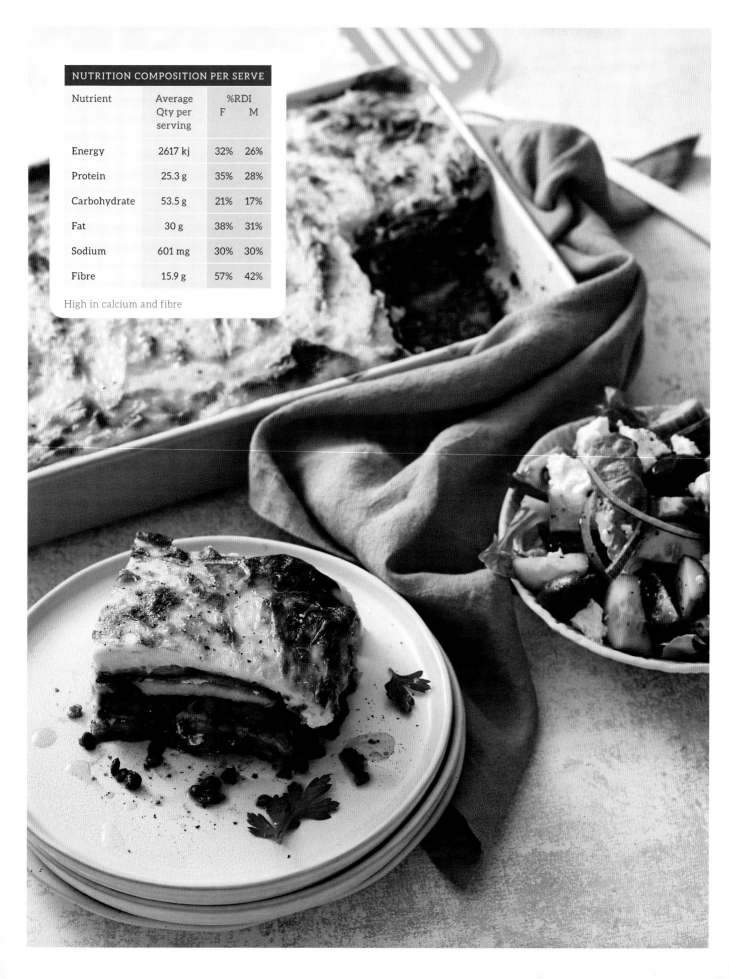

NUTRITION COMPOSITION PER SERVE			
Nutrient	Average Qty per serving	%RDI F	M
Energy	2617 kj	32%	26%
Protein	25.3 g	35%	28%
Carbohydrate	53.5 g	21%	17%
Fat	30 g	38%	31%
Sodium	601 mg	30%	30%
Fibre	15.9 g	57%	42%

High in calcium and fibre

Vegetarian moussaka
with lentil bolognese

⅓ cup (80 ml) extra-virgin olive oil,
plus extra for frying

1 red onion, finely chopped

1–2 garlic cloves, finely chopped

1 small red chilli, halved, deseeded and
finely chopped

4–5 Swiss brown mushrooms, cleaned
and quartered

4 large eggplants, 1 roughly diced and
3 sliced lengthways (5 mm thick)

3 x 400 g tins lentils, drained and rinsed

½ cup (125 ml) red wine

1 x 400 g tin chopped tomatoes

1 cup (250 ml) puréed tomato

1 cup (250 ml) boiling water, plus extra
if needed

3 tablespoons chopped flat-leaf parsley

Sea salt and freshly ground black pepper

3 large potatoes, sliced (5 mm thick)

200 g feta

Greek salad, to serve

BECHAMEL SAUCE

100 g butter

100 g plain flour

4 cups (1 litre) milk

My daughter Tiana has inherited the ability to quickly fry up kilos of eggplants and potatoes and assemble this family favourite. Getting the family involved is the best way to cook!

Heat some olive oil in a large frying pan over a medium heat and sauté the onion until softened and translucent. Add the garlic and chilli and continue to cook for a few minutes, taking care not to burn the garlic.

Meanwhile, place the mushroom and the diced eggplant in a food processor and pulse until finely minced. Add this to the onion mixture and sauté for 10 minutes.

Add the lentils and red wine to the pan and cook until the alcohol evaporates. Add the tinned and puréed tomatoes and boiling water. Simmer for 20 minutes to thicken, ensuring the mixture does not dry out too much – add extra boiling water as needed. Add 2 tablespoons of parsley for the last 5 minutes of cooking and season with salt and pepper to taste. Remove from the heat and set aside.

Heat some olive oil in a large heavy-based frying pan and fry the eggplant and potato slices on both sides until golden. Transfer to a plate lined with kitchen paper to drain. If you prefer to use less oil, brush the vegetables lightly with olive oil and chargrill on a hotplate or under the grill.

Preheat the oven to 180°C. Assemble the moussaka by spreading a little of the lentil bolognese around the base of a large baking dish, then follow with a layer of potato slices. Spoon over a 1 cm thick layer of lentil bolognese, then crumble on some feta and sprinkle over some parsley. Add a layer of eggplant, then repeat with the bolognese, feta and parsley – alternating between the potato and eggplant layers until all the ingredients are finished.

Melt the butter for the bechamel in a heavy-based saucepan over a medium heat. Whisk in the flour to make a roux. Gradually add the milk and whisk well to prevent lumps from forming. Cook, stirring, until the bechamel resembles custard. Season with salt and pepper.

Spread the bechamel on top of the moussaka and bake for 30–45 minutes, or until lightly browned on top. Allow to cool for 10 minutes, slice into 4 cm squares and serve with a Greek salad.

Vegan lentil shepherd's pie

COOKING 2 HOURS

SERVES 8

3 large eggplants, 1 roughly diced,
  2 sliced lengthways (5 mm thick)

3 large zucchini, sliced lengthways
  (5 mm thick)

⅓ cup (80 ml) extra-virgin olive oil,
  plus extra for brushing

1 red onion, finely chopped

1–2 garlic cloves, finely chopped

Optional: 1 small green chilli, halved,
  deseeded and finely chopped

⅓ cup (45 g) crushed macadamia nuts
  (see tip)

300 g Swiss brown mushrooms, quartered

2 x 400 g tins brown lentils, drained
  and rinsed

½ cup (125 ml) red wine

500 g tomatoes, grated (see tip on
  page 97) or 300 ml purèed tomato

2 tablespoons tomato paste

½ teaspoon smoked paprika

1 cup (250 ml) boiling water, plus extra
  if needed

½ bunch basil, leaves picked

Salad, to serve

POTATO BECHAMEL

600 g potatoes (low-carbohydrate
  potatoes such as carisma if possible),
  peeled and roughly diced

50 g dairy-free margarine

200 ml soy, oat, almond or rice milk,
  heated

2–3 tablespoons macadamia cream
  (see tip)

Sea salt and freshly ground black pepper

Pinch ground nutmeg

This hearty dish combines vegetarian moussaka ingredients to create a vegan version of a classic Irish dish.

To make the potato bechamel, cook the potatoes in salted boiling water for 20 minutes or until soft, then mash. Beat the margarine, soy milk and macadamia cream into the potatoes until creamy. Season with salt and pepper to taste and nutmeg, then set aside.

Heat a hotplate or chargrill pan over a medium heat. Brush the eggplant and zucchini slices with olive oil, chargrill until soft and set aside.

Heat some olive oil in a large flameproof casserole dish over a medium heat and sauté the onion until softened and translucent. Add the garlic and chilli (if using) and sauté for a few minutes, taking care not to burn the garlic.

Meanwhile, place the mushroom and diced eggplant in a food processor and pulse until finely chopped. Add to the onion mixture and sauté for 10–15 minutes.

Add the lentils and red wine to the dish, and cook until the alcohol evaporates. Next, add the grated or puréed tomato, tomato paste, paprika and boiling water. Simmer for 20 minutes until thickened, ensuring the bolognese does not dry out too much. Add extra boiling water if needed. Tear in half the basil leaves in the last 5 minutes of cooking, then season with salt and pepper to taste. Set aside.

Preheat the oven to 180°C. Assemble the moussaka in a large baking dish. Start by spreading a layer of lentil bolognese on the base of the dish, then cover with a layer of eggplant slices. Add another 1 cm thick layer of lentil bolognese and some basil. Follow with a layer of zucchini slices. Repeat the layering, alternating between the zucchini and eggplant layers until all the ingredients are used. Set aside.

Spread the potato bechamel on top of the moussaka, then bake for 45 minutes, or until lightly browned on top. Allow to cool for a few minutes before slicing into eight even portions. Serve with a Greek or green salad.

TIPS

Adding ⅓ cup (45 g) crushed macadamia nuts, walnuts or pine nuts to the lentil mushroom bolognese adds crunch to the dish and makes the sauce richer in flavour. And adding 2–3 tablespoons of macadamia cream to the bechamel when beating the milk in adds richness to the flavour and creaminess to the sauce.

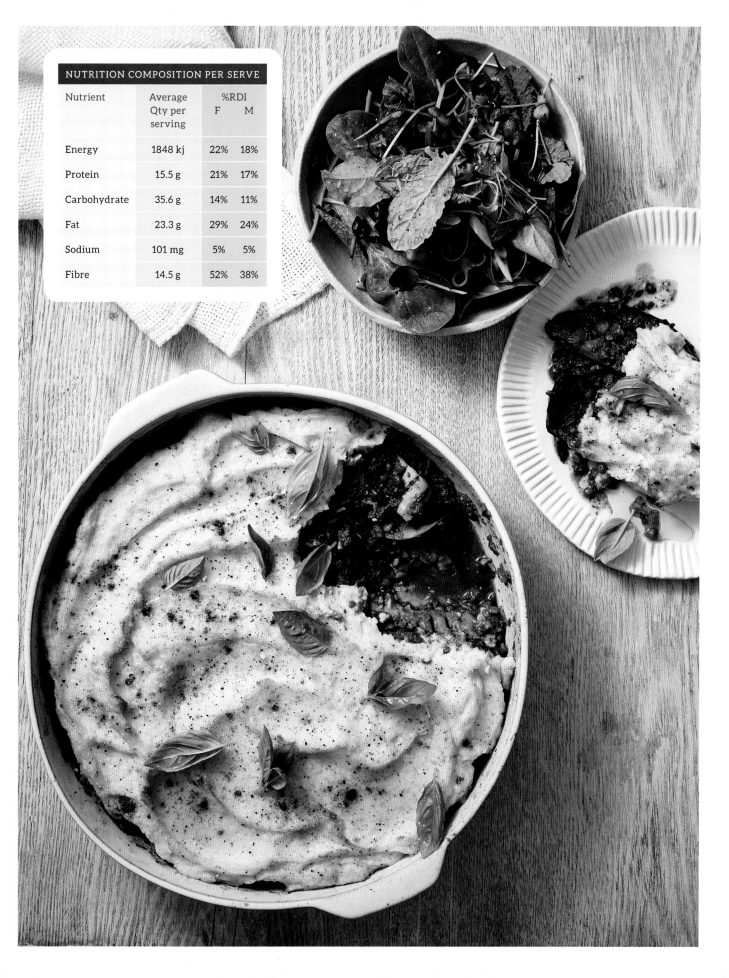

NUTRITION COMPOSITION PER SERVE			
Nutrient	Average Qty per serving	%RDI F	M
Energy	1848 kj	22%	18%
Protein	15.5 g	21%	17%
Carbohydrate	35.6 g	14%	11%
Fat	23.3 g	29%	24%
Sodium	101 mg	5%	5%
Fibre	14.5 g	52%	38%

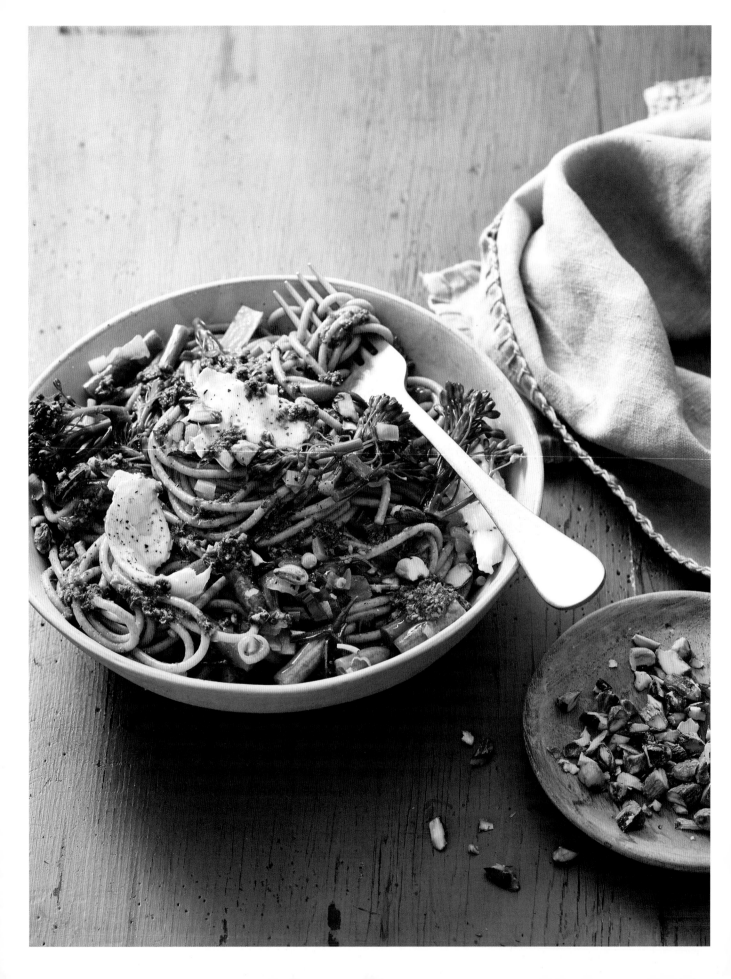

Spaghetti with spring vegetables and pesto

COOKING
15
MINUTES

SERVES
4

2 tablespoons extra-virgin olive oil

1 onion, finely chopped

1 long red chilli, halved, deseeded
   and sliced

1 bunch broccolini, cut into 2 cm lengths

200 g green beans, blanched and cut
   into 2 cm lengths

1 bunch spring onions, finely chopped

4 tablespoons Traditional basil pesto
   (see page 84)

Sea salt and freshly ground black pepper

500 g spaghetti

Optional: 1 x 150 g ball buffalo mozzarella
   or fresh ricotta

1 tablespoon crushed pistachios

This pesto pasta with spring greens was inspired by a dish
I enjoyed at a local Italian restaurant. Bellissimo!

Heat the olive oil in a large deep frying pan and sauté the onion until
softened and translucent. Add the chilli, broccolini and green beans,
and stir until the beans are slightly softened. Add the spring onion and
pesto, then stir and season with salt and pepper to taste.

Meanwhile, boil the spaghetti in salted water and cook until al dente,
then drain, reserving ½ cup (125 ml) of the pasta cooking water.

Add the pasta to the pan and toss through, adding some of the
reserved cooking water if needed (you want this to be quite runny
and not too dry).

Divide between four pasta bowls and add a few slices of buffalo
mozzarella or dollops of ricotta (if using), drizzle with olive oil, season
with pepper, then sprinkle with the pistachios and serve.

NUTRITION COMPOSITION PER SERVE			
Nutrient	Average Qty per serving	%RDI F	M
Energy	2307 kj	28%	23%
Protein	18.5 g	25%	21%
Carbohydrate	65.5 g	26%	20%
Fat	22.5 g	28%	23%
Sodium	101 mg	5%	5%
Fibre	14.5 g	52%	38%

High in calcium, if adding cheese, and in fibre

Harvest pie

2 sheets puff pastry (see note)

Extra-virgin olive oil

1 onion, finely chopped

1 leek, white and light green parts only,
 finely sliced and washed

1 garlic clove, finely chopped

1 celery stalk, chopped

1 cup roughly chopped wild greens
 such as amaranth, sow thistle,
 dandelion or silverbeet

2–3 flat-leaf parsley sprigs, leaves picked
 and chopped, plus extra to serve

2–3 dill fronds, chopped, plus extra
 to serve

2–3 mint sprigs, leaves picked and
 chopped, plus extra to serve

2–3 basil sprigs, leaves picked and
 chopped, plus extra to serve

150 g baby zucchini, sliced in half
 lengthways or 2–3 zucchini flowers,
 sliced in half lengthways

Optional: 100 g baby eggplants, sliced
 lengthways

100 g fresh ricotta

100 g feta

Sea salt and freshly ground black pepper

Lemon wedges, if on hand

Green salad and/or Beetroot, tahini and
 yoghurt dip, to serve

My daughter Vivienne and her friend Juliet love to create vegetarian dishes like this delicious pie with Mediterranean vegetables and plenty of fresh herbs.

Preheat the oven to 180°C. Line a large roasting tin with baking paper, then lay the sheets of puff pastry next to each other in the tin so the base of the tin is completely covered.

Heat 2 tablespoons of olive oil in a large frying pan and sauté the onion until softened and translucent. Add the leek, garlic and celery and continue to cook for a few minutes until the leek begins to soften.

Add the greens and fresh herbs to the pan and cook until they are wilted, then spoon and spread the vegetable mixture over the puff pastry, leaving a 3 cm border around the edges. Fold the pastry sides in and brush lightly with olive oil.

Return the frying pan to the heat, add a little olive oil and fry the zucchini and eggplant (if using) on both sides, then arrange over the vegetable mixture. If using zucchini flowers, add them now.

Dot the cheeses all over the pie, alternating between the ricotta and feta. Season with salt and pepper to taste, then bake for 30 minutes, taking care not to burn the greens.

Scatter over the extra herbs before serving with a lemon wedge, if on hand, a leafy green salad and/or the Beetroot, tahini and yoghurt dip (see page 112).

NOTE

You can make this pie gluten-free if you can track down a good-quality gluten-free puff pastry.

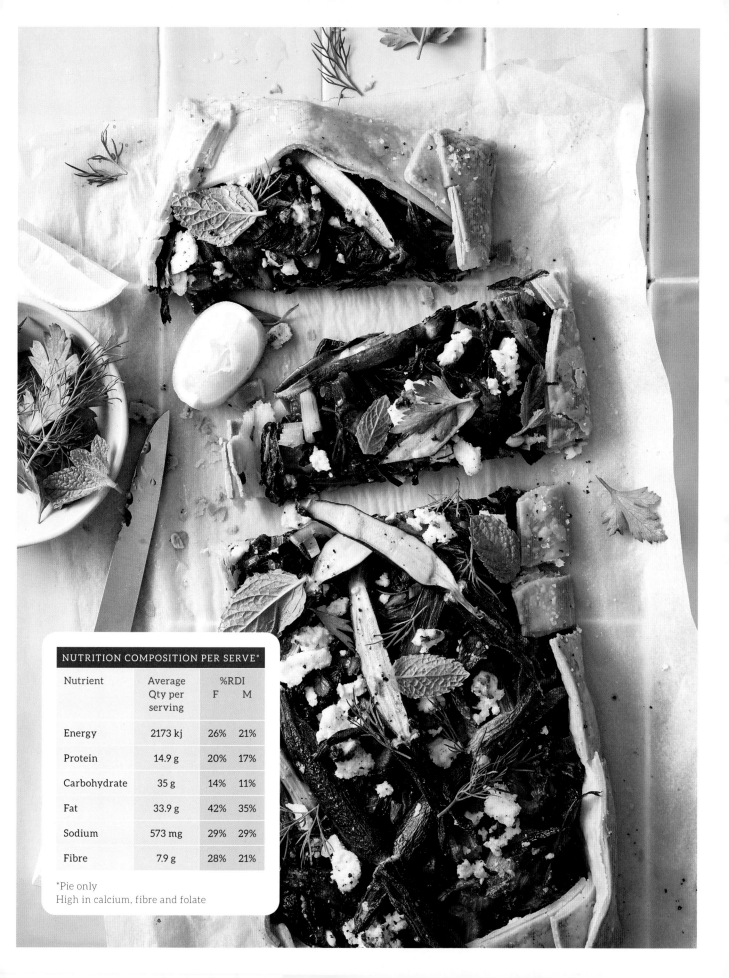

NUTRITION COMPOSITION PER SERVE*

Nutrient	Average Qty per serving	%RDI F	M
Energy	2173 kj	26%	21%
Protein	14.9 g	20%	17%
Carbohydrate	35 g	14%	11%
Fat	33.9 g	42%	35%
Sodium	573 mg	29%	29%
Fibre	7.9 g	28%	21%

*Pie only
High in calcium, fibre and folate

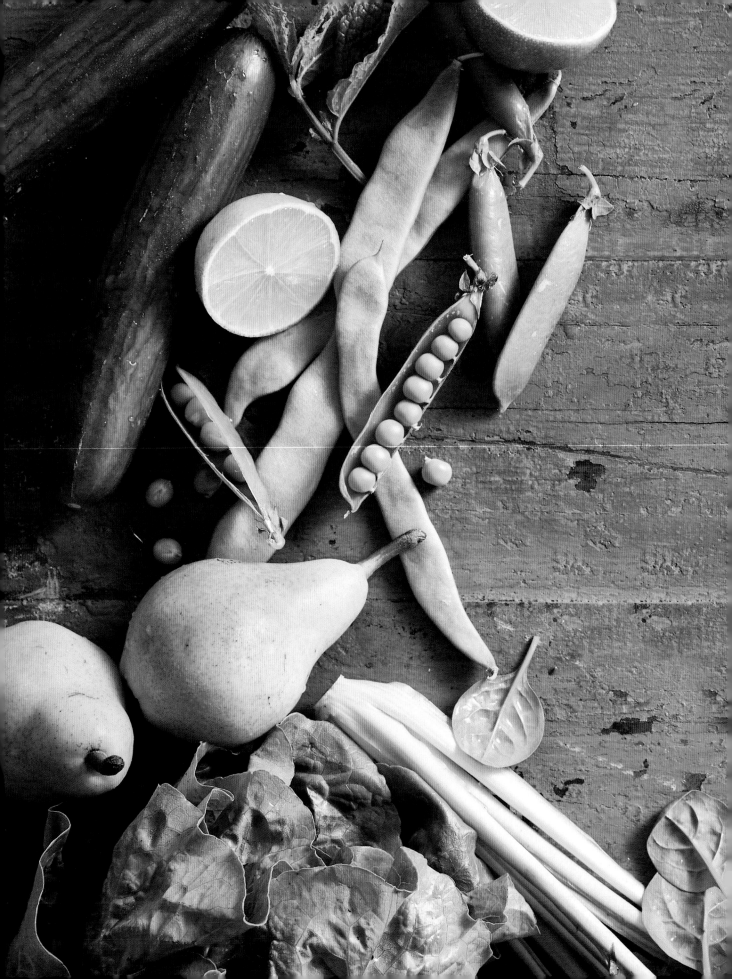

Soups
and
salads

—

Zucchini tagliatelle salad
with chilli and pistachios

2 large (about 300 g) zucchini, cut into
   long, wide strips using a peeler,
   vegetable slicer or Asian grater

½ fennel bulb, finely sliced, plus fronds

1 small red chilli, halved, deseeded
   and finely sliced

1 tablespoon roughly chopped pistachios

2 tablespoons extra-virgin olive oil

Juice 1 lemon

Fresh herbs, if on hand

Sea salt and freshly ground black pepper

Eat more greens with this fresh zucchini salad marinated
with extra-virgin olive oil, lemon juice and fresh chillies.

Arrange the strips of zucchini in a serving dish, then scatter the
fennel slices, chilli and pistachios on top.

Dress with the olive oil and lemon juice, sprinkle over the fennel
fronds, garnish with the fresh herbs, if on hand, and season with
salt and pepper to taste, then serve.

NUTRITION COMPOSITION PER SERVE			
Nutrient	Average Qty per serving	%RDI F	M
Energy	270 kj	3%	3%
Protein	1 g	1%	1%
Carbohydrate	2.6 g	1%	1%
Fat	5 g	6%	5%
Sodium	51 mg	3%	3%
Fibre	2 g	7%	5%

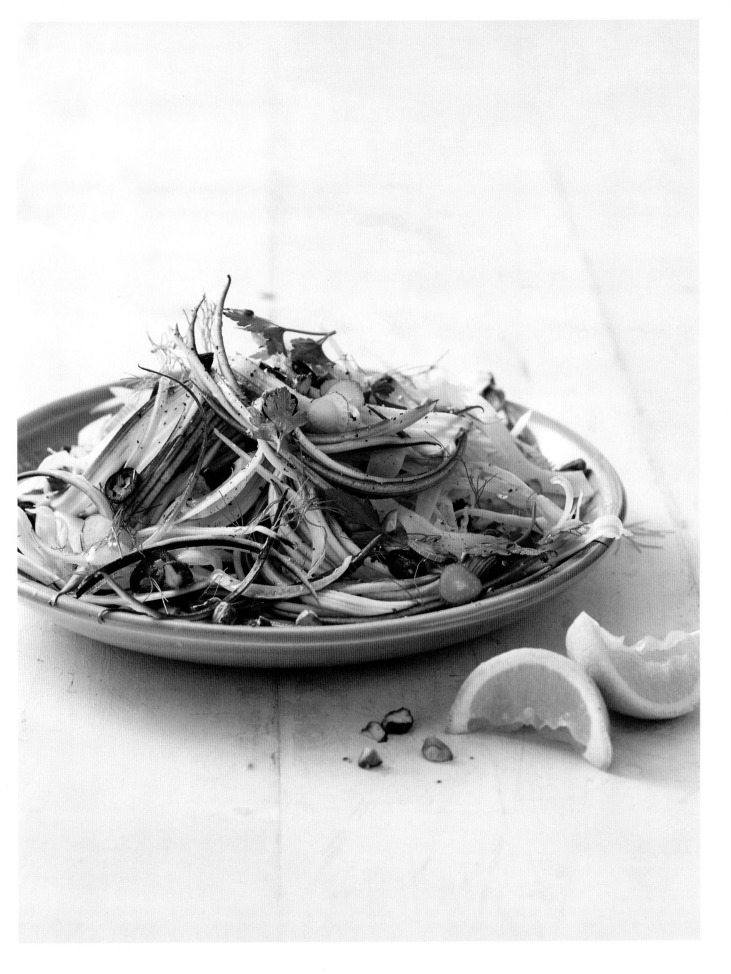

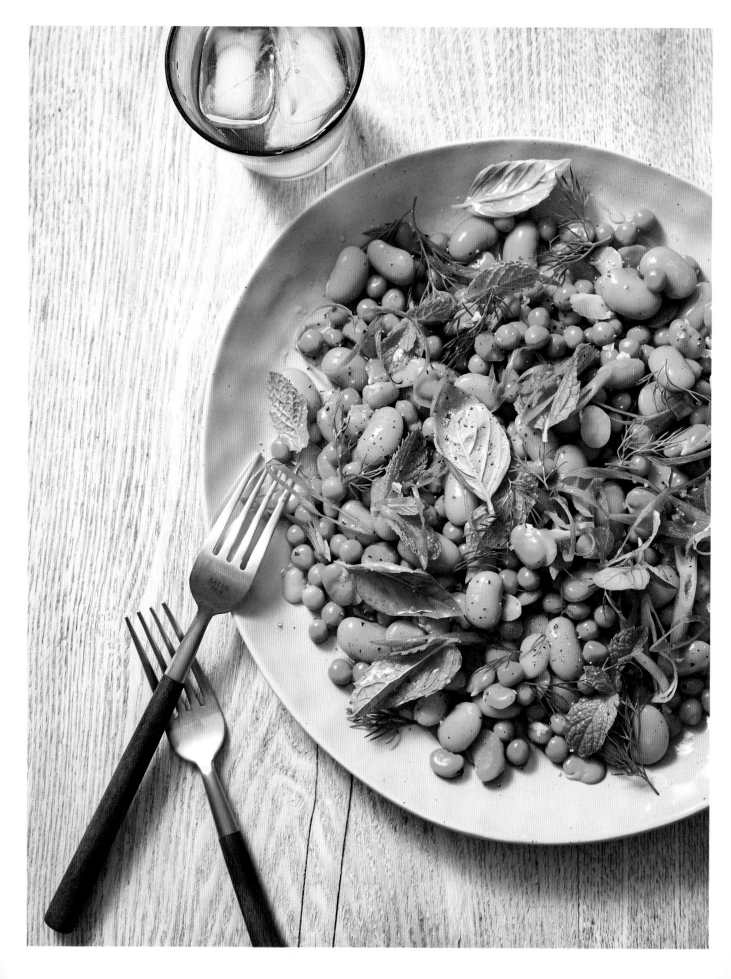

Warm *broad bean* and pea salad

SERVES 6 AS A SIDE

500 g podded broad beans (fresh or frozen)

500 g peas (fresh or frozen)

2 tablespoons finely chopped chives

2 tablespoons finely chopped dill

2 tablespoons finely chopped mint leaves

Sea salt and freshly ground black pepper

¼ cup (60 ml) extra-virgin olive oil

50 g butter, melted

Juice 1 lemon

2 tablespoons basil leaves

Optional: 1 tablespoon grated parmesan

Peas, beans and greens are always on hand to make this impressive warm salad inspired by my daughter Vivienne. Just add fresh herbs and dress liberally with extra-virgin olive oil and fresh lemon juice. For a more decadent dish, try adding creamy stracciatella or burrata.

If the broad beans are frozen, soak them in cold water for 10 minutes before peeling off their skins, then blanch. If fresh, boil the peas for 10 minutes until soft, or blanch if frozen.

Put the peas and broad beans on a serving platter. Add the finely chopped herbs and season with salt and pepper to taste.

Mix the olive oil, melted butter and lemon juice together, then dress the salad and top with the basil leaves and parmesan (if using).

TIP

For a more decadent salad, spread the base of a serving platter with 250 g fresh ricotta whipped with the zest and juice of ½ lemon and seasoned with salt and pepper to taste. Arrange the tossed bean salad over the top.

NUTRITION COMPOSITION PER SERVE			
Nutrient	Average Qty per serving	%RDI F	M
Energy	871 kj	11%	8%
Protein	10.3 g	14%	11%
Carbohydrate	12.4 g	5%	4%
Fat	10.1 g	13%	10%
Sodium	252 mg	13%	13%
Fibre	11.4 g	41%	30%

High in fibre and folate

SOUPS AND SALADS   137

Poached pear and fig salad with caramelised walnuts

COOKING **30** MINUTES

SERVES **2**

POACHED PEARS

2 brown or green pears, quartered

1½ cups (375 ml) sweet white wine, such as moscato

Ground nutmeg

SALAD

1 x 60 g bag of mixed lettuce leaves

Small handful of rocket leaves

200 g broccolini

1 tablespoon pitted kalamata olives

2 tablespoons toasted or caramelised walnuts (see page 155)

4 fresh figs, quartered

2 tablespoons extra-virgin olive oil

2 tablespoons apple cider vinegar

Sea salt and freshly ground black pepper

20 g blue cheese, crumbled

A modern Mediterranean salad that combines fresh figs, poached pears and leafy greens, topped with caramelised walnuts that are rich in plant omega-3 fats. This salad works best assembled on individual plates.

Put the pears and wine in a saucepan over a high heat. Add a few pinches of nutmeg, then bring to the boil. Once boiling, reduce the heat to low and simmer for 30 minutes. Carefully remove the pears using a slotted spoon and set aside.

Divide the salad leaves, broccolini, olives, walnuts and figs between two serving plates. Arrange the poached pears on top of each salad, then drizzle with the olive oil and apple cider vinegar, and season with salt and pepper to taste. Crumble the blue cheese on top before serving.

NUTRITION COMPOSITION PER SERVE			
Nutrient	Average Qty per serving	%RDI F	M
Energy	2203 kj	27%	21%
Protein	11.5 g	16%	13%
Carbohydrate	36.9 g	15%	12%
Fat	26.4 g	33%	27%
Sodium	302 mg	15%	15%
Fibre	15.2 g	54%	40%

High in fibre, folate and b-carotene

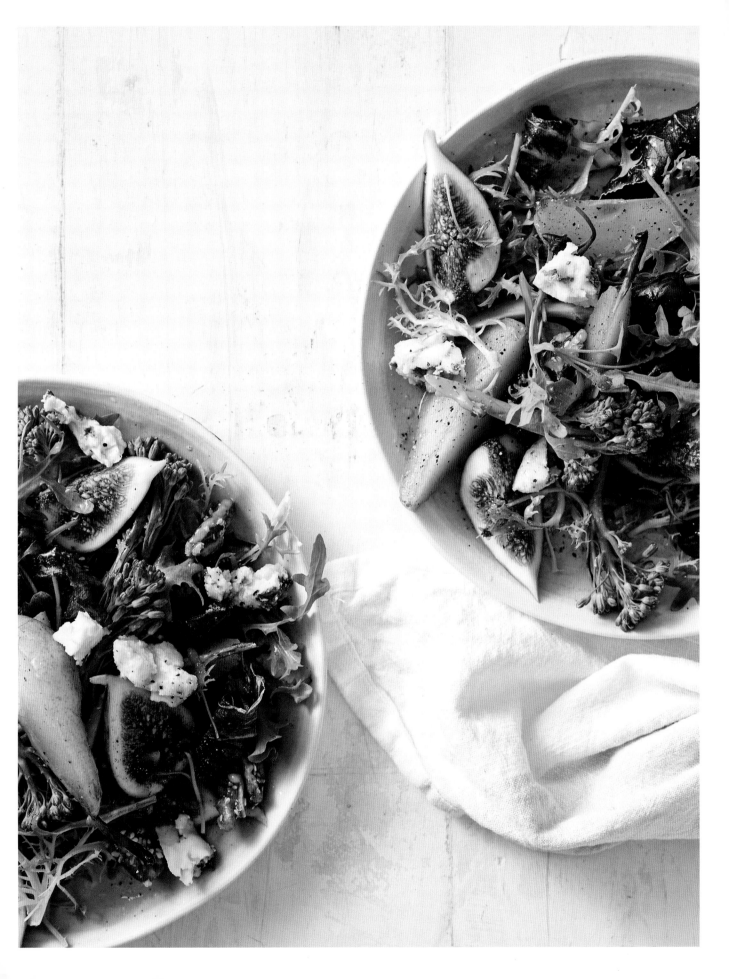

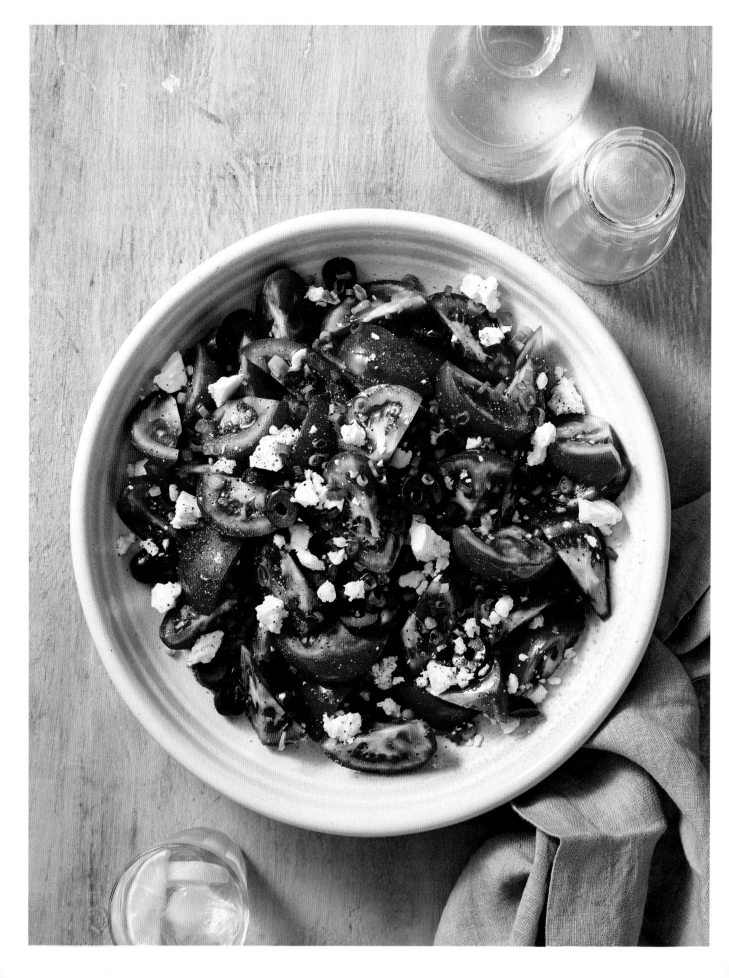

Fresh *tomato* salad

400 g vine-ripened tomatoes,
    roughly chopped

2 tablespoons pitted kalamata olives,
    sliced

½ bunch spring onions, finely chopped

60 g feta, crumbled

2 tablespoons extra-virgin olive oil

Sea salt and freshly ground black pepper

Optional: drizzle of balsamic glaze,
    to serve

In-season vine-ripened tomatoes are meant to be enjoyed with simple dressings. This salad works well with the Spicy lamb ribs on page 196.

Combine the tomato, olives, sping onion, feta and olive oil in a salad bowl, toss together, then season with salt and pepper to taste. Drizzle with the balsamic glaze before serving, if you like.

NUTRITION COMPOSITION PER SERVE			
Nutrient	Average Qty per serving	%RDI F	M
Energy	630 kj	8%	6%
Protein	3.6 g	5%	4%
Carbohydrate	3.3 g	1%	1%
Fat	13.4 g	17%	14%
Sodium	269 mg	13%	13%
Fibre	1.2 g	4%	3%

Pickling *olives*

1 kg uncured kalamata olives
 or other fresh olives

BRINE

3 cups (750 ml) boiling water

1 cup cooking salt

1 egg

1 lemon, halved

1 cup (250 ml) white vinegar

Extra-virgin olive oil

FLAVOUR OPTIONS
(TO YOUR TASTE)

Sliced green chillies (can also use red)
 to taste or 2 teaspoons chilli flakes

1 tablespoon picked thyme leaves

1 tablespoon chopped rosemary

1 tablespoon capers

4–5 peeled garlic cloves

You'll need a 1 litre capacity pickling jar
 with a lid

A Mediterranean table is not complete without olives. Rich in monounsaturated fats and polyphenols and with a great salty taste, olives are the perfect accompaniment to any meal with a glass of red wine.

Step 1: Start by 'debittering' the olives. Use a small, sharp knife to make a small incision lengthways in each olive. Wash well, then place in a large jar with a lid. Fill with water and leave for one week, replacing the water daily.

Step 2: Make a brine by mixing the boiling water and salt together in a large container. Cool in the refrigerator for a few hours. To test the salt concentration, place the egg in the brine; if it floats, the salinity is correct. If it doesn't float, mix in another tablespoon of salt, then test again.

Step 3: Drain the olives and replace the water in the jar with the prepared brine.

Step 4: Add the halved lemon to the jar along with any of the flavourings listed. Top with the white vinegar, then put the lid on and shake to mix well. Pour in enough olive oil to cover the olives by at least 2 cm – this will prevent mould from growing.

Step 5: Seal and store the olives in a dark, cool place for at least 6 weeks to cure.

Step 6: These olives can be served straight from the brine, or stored in smaller jars and marinated in olive oil with the flavourings of your choice. These will keep for one year or more. Once opened, store in the refrigerator.

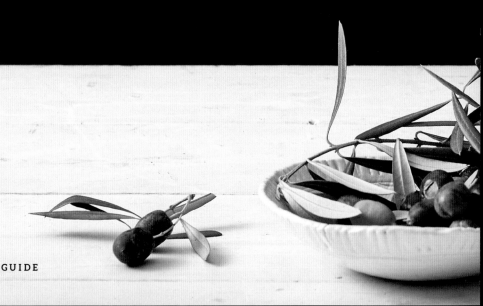

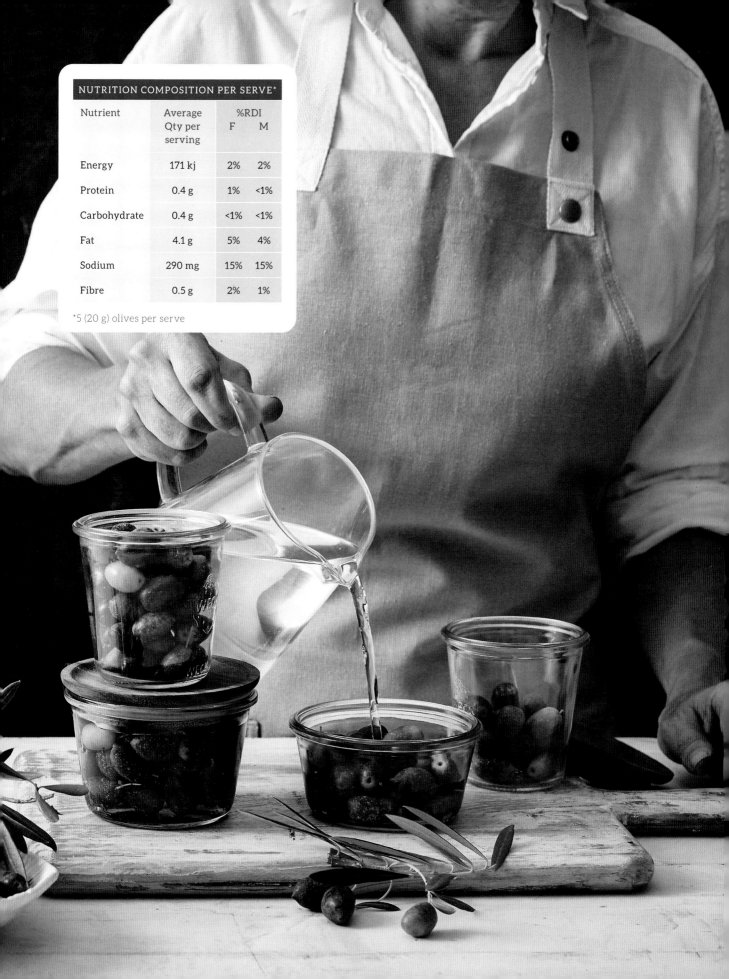

NUTRITION COMPOSITION PER SERVE*

Nutrient	Average Qty per serving	%RDI F	M
Energy	171 kj	2%	2%
Protein	0.4 g	1%	<1%
Carbohydrate	0.4 g	<1%	<1%
Fat	4.1 g	5%	4%
Sodium	290 mg	15%	15%
Fibre	0.5 g	2%	1%

*5 (20 g) olives per serve

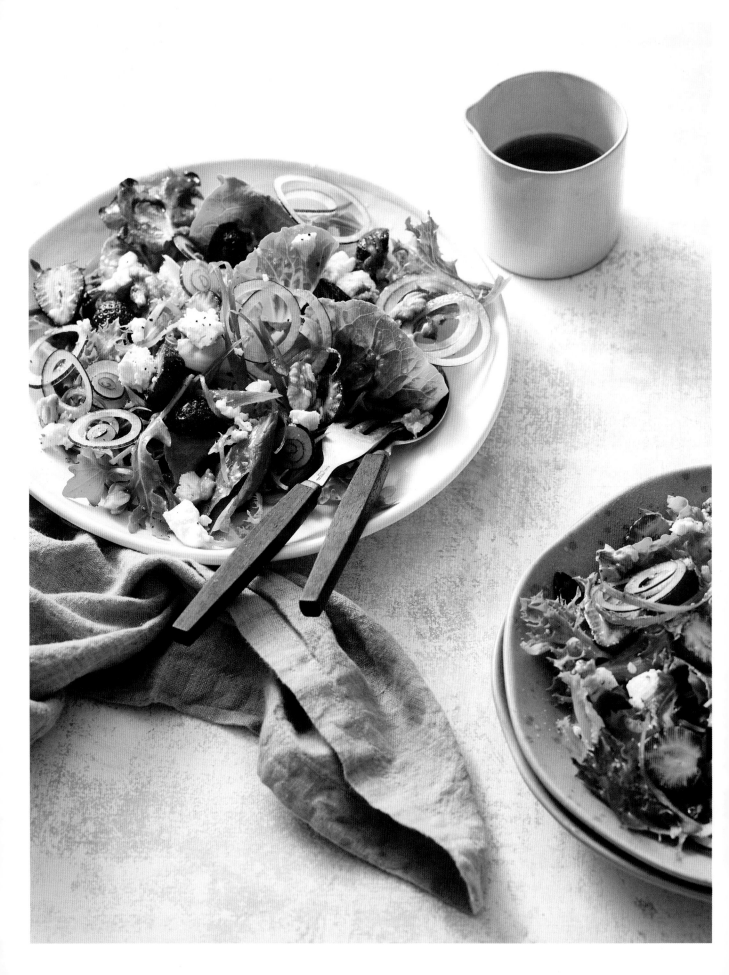

Seychelles salad

SERVES

2

AS A SIDE

4 handfuls mixed green salad leaves

½ punnet (125 g) strawberries, hulled
   and halved

1 small red onion, finely sliced

4 spring onions, finely chopped

2 tablespoons toasted or caramelised
   walnuts (see page 155)

60 g manouri cheese, finely sliced, or
   goat's cheese, crumbled

DRESSING

2 tablespoons extra-virgin olive oil

2 tablespoons white balsamic vinegar
   or white wine vinegar

Sea salt and freshly ground black pepper

This salad is named after one of my favourite 'edgy'
restaurants in Athens, which specialises in mezze and ouzo.
This recipe combines sweet strawberries with sharp goat's
cheese and works well with pasta dishes or moussaka.

Put all the dressing ingredients in a small jar with a lid and shake
together to mix.

Place all the salad ingredients except the cheese in a serving bowl.
Drizzle over the dressing, then gently toss. Add the slices of manouri
cheese or crumbled goat's cheese on top before serving.

NUTRITION COMPOSITION PER SERVE			
Nutrient	Average Qty per serving	%RDI F	M
Energy	850 kj	10%	8%
Protein	5.1 g	7%	6%
Carbohydrate	11.1 g	4%	3%
Fat	14.9 g	19%	15%
Sodium	118 mg	6%	6%
Fibre	2.7 g	10%	7%

SOUPS AND SALADS   145

Green bean salad with flaked almonds and peaches

COOKING
10
MINUTES

SERVES
4
AS A SIDE

400 g green beans, trimmed
and halved lengthways

1 tablespoon extra-virgin olive oil

Juice ½ lemon

Sea salt and freshly ground black pepper

1 yellow peach, sliced

1 tablespoon crushed, toasted or flaked
almonds

Fresh herbs, if on hand

Combining fresh in-season peaches with green beans gives this salad a great sweet and savoury contrast. Try using brown pears when peaches are not in season.

Boil the beans in a saucepan over a medium heat for 10 minutes, or until they are just soft, take care not to overcook them. Drain the beans, then transfer to a serving bowl or platter. Dress with the olive oil and lemon juice and season with salt and pepper to taste.

Just before serving, top the salad with the peach slices and almonds and garnish with the fresh herbs, if on hand.

Nutrient	Average Qty per serving	%RDI F	M
NUTRITION COMPOSITION PER SERVE			
Energy	436 kj	5%	4%
Protein	2.8 g	4%	3%
Carbohydrate	7.6 g	3%	2%
Fat	10 g	13%	10%
Sodium	39 mg	2%	2%
Fibre	4.3 g	15%	11%

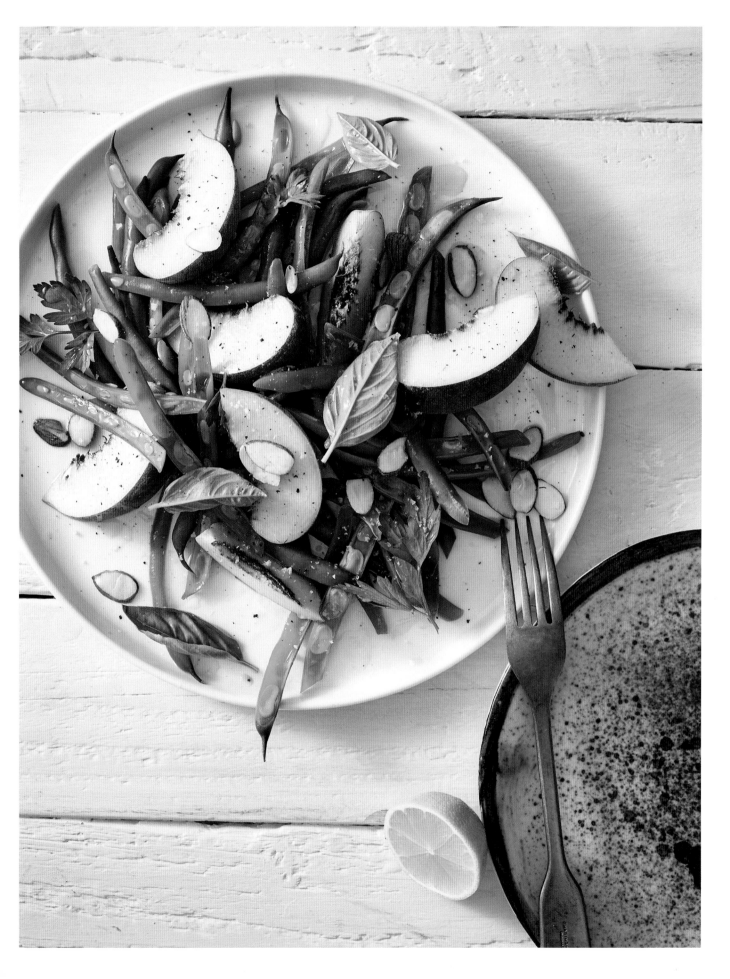

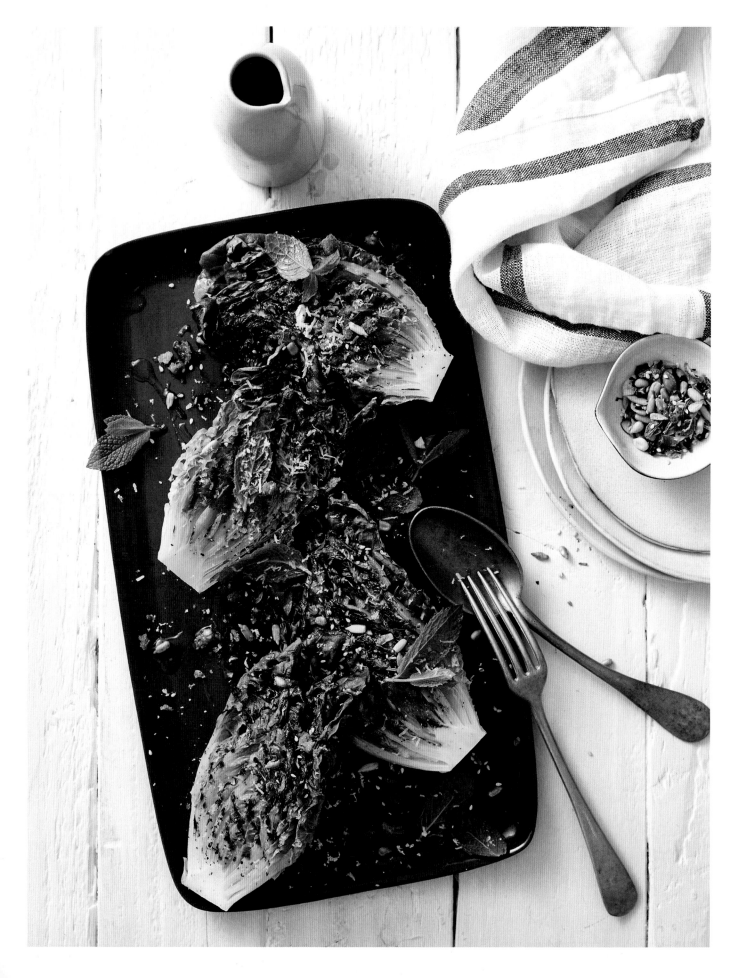

Chargrilled cos with pangrattato and grated cheese

COOKING
10
MINUTES

SERVES
2

1 tablespoon extra-virgin olive oil,
  plus extra for frying

1 tablespoon gluten-free breadcrumbs

Freshly ground black pepper

1 tablespoon mixed seeds, lightly toasted

2 baby cos lettuces, washed and halved
  lengthways

20 g mizithra cheese or parmesan, grated

Fresh herbs, if on hand

Lightly charred cos lettuce topped with toasted seeds and pangrattato (breadcrumbs) goes well with the grilled pork cutlets on page 212.

Heat a drizzle of olive oil in a small frying pan over a medium heat. Add the breadcrumbs and fry for a few minutes with a pinch of pepper until evenly golden and crisp. Transfer to a plate and allow to cool.

Return the pan to the heat and lightly toast the mixed seeds for a few minutes, then remove from the heat.

Heat a chargrill pan over a medium–high heat and add the remaining olive oil. Place the lettuce halves, cut-side down, on the pan and chargrill for a few minutes, until the side touching the pan is lightly browned but not wilted.

Place the lettuce halves, cut-side up, on a serving plate and sprinkle over the toasted seeds and pangrattato, then top with the grated cheese and garnish with the fresh herbs, if on hand. Serve right away.

NUTRITION COMPOSITION PER SERVE			
Nutrient	Average Qty per serving	%RDI F	M
Energy	937 kj	11%	9%
Protein	8 g	11%	9%
Carbohydrate	7.7 g	3%	2%
Fat	17.5 g	22%	18%
Sodium	207 mg	10%	10%
Fibre	2.5 g	9%	7%

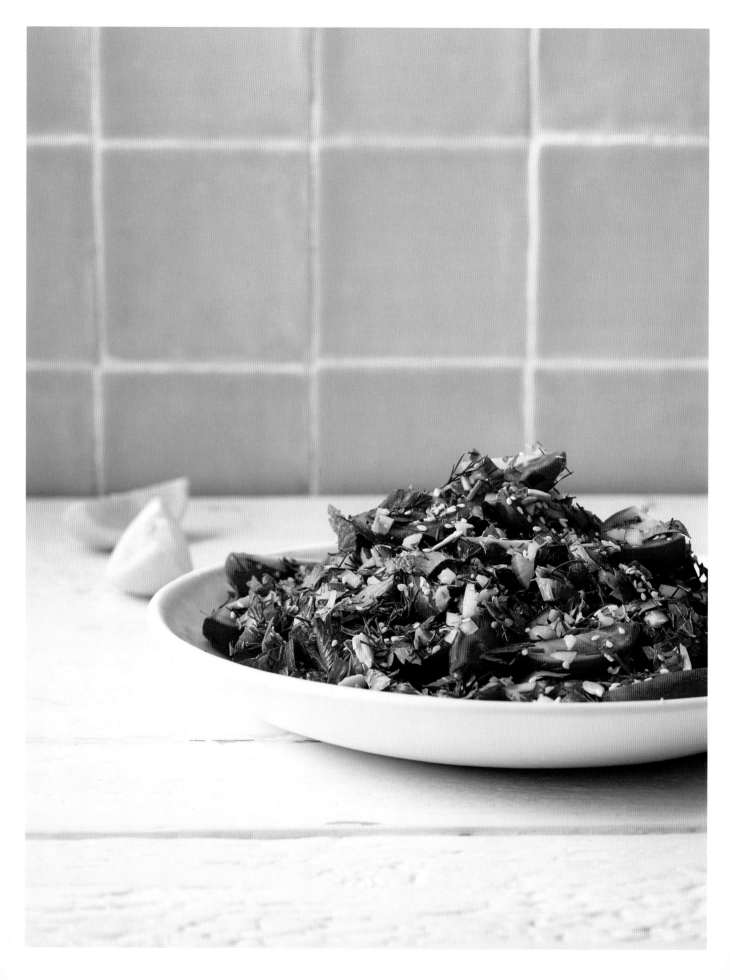

Chickpea tabbouleh

1 bunch of flat-leaf parsley, roughly
  chopped

2 tablespoons chopped dill

2 tablespoons chopped mint

1 small red onion, finely diced

1 punnet (250 g) baby roma tomatoes,
  quartered

2 tablespoons crushed chickpeas
  (soak ½ cup (100 g) dried chickpeas
  overnight, then drain and roughly chop
  in a food processor)

1 tablespoon toasted mixed seeds

2–3 tablespoons extra-virgin olive oil

Juice 1 lemon

Sea salt and freshly ground black pepper

Tabbouleh is a traditional Lebanese salad made with parsley and bulgur or cracked wheat. In this recipe I have varied the herbs and created a gluten-free option with chickpeas instead of bulgur. You will need to begin this recipe a day ahead.

Mix all the ingredients together in a large serving bowl and serve as a side dish or as a filling for souvlaki (see page 205).

NUTRITION COMPOSITION PER SERVE			
Nutrient	Average Qty per serving	%RDI F	M
Energy	505 kj	6%	5%
Protein	2.6 g	4%	3%
Carbohydrate	3.8 g	2%	1%
Fat	9.8 g	12%	10%
Sodium	44 mg	2%	2%
Fibre	3.6 g	13%	9%

Citrus and fennel salad

2 oranges

Optional: 1 blood orange or 1 Cara Cara
   orange

2 honey murcott mandarins

1 pink grapefruit

Juice 2 limes

½ fennel bulb, plus fronds

1 small red onion

1–2 tablespoons flaked almonds

1 tablespoon finely chopped mint, plus
   extra leaves to serve

Extra-virgin olive oil

Sea salt and freshly ground black pepper

This vibrant citrus salad is rich in vitamin C and is a typical dish of Spanish and Sicilian cuisines.

Peel the oranges, mandarins and grapefruit, then carefully slice them into rounds using a sharp knife. Arrange these rounds in a shallow salad bowl, then squeeze the lime juice over the top.

Finely slice the fennel lengthways and scatter over the citrus. Finely slice the red onion and scatter over the salad. Sprinkle over the flaked almonds, mint and fennel fronds, then dress with a drizzle of olive oil. Season with salt and pepper to taste, then serve.

NUTRITION COMPOSITION PER SERVE			
Nutrient	Average Qty per serving	%RDI F	M
Energy	751 kj	9%	7%
Protein	3.6 g	5%	4%
Carbohydrate	17.9 g	7%	6%
Fat	8.8 g	11%	9%
Sodium	38.8 mg	2%	2%
Fibre	6.3 g	23%	17%

High in vitamin C

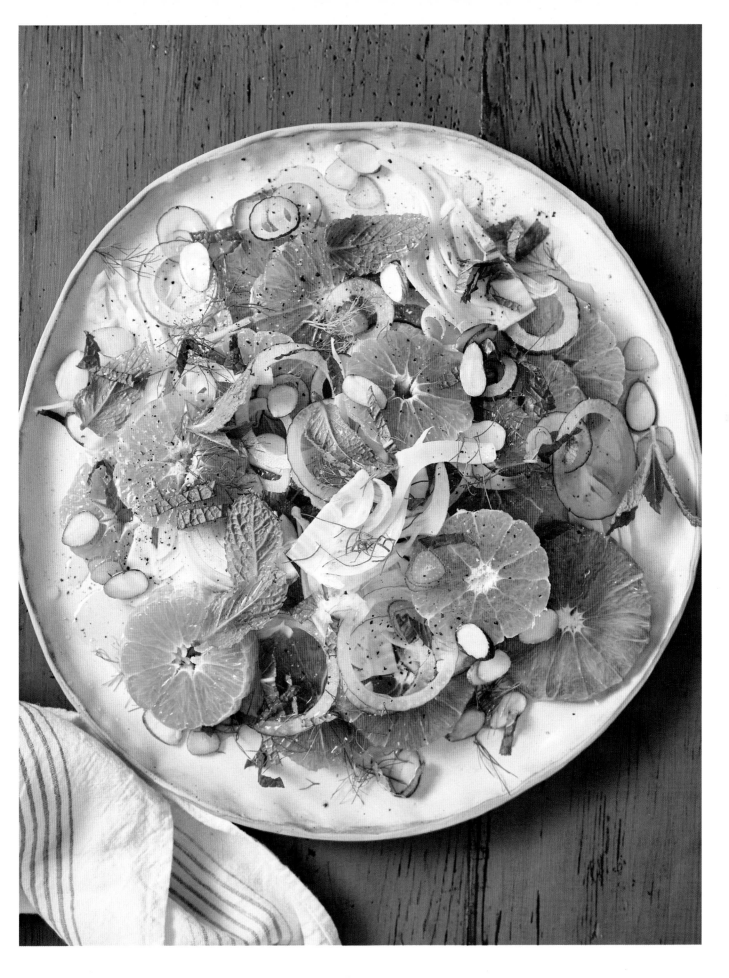

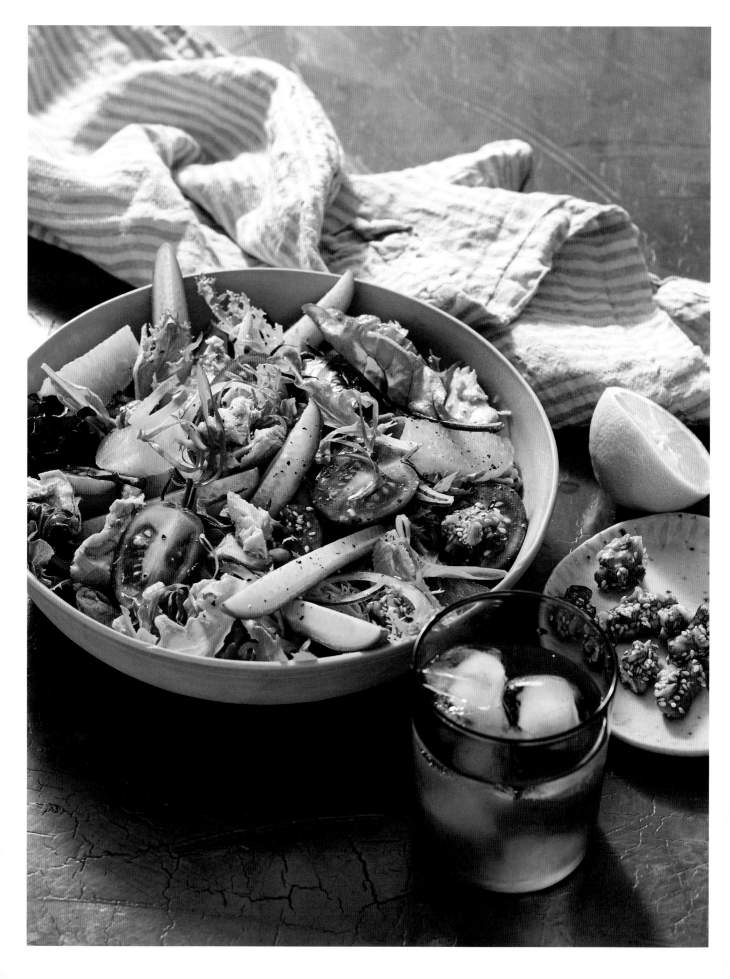

Salmon and orange salad with caramelised walnuts

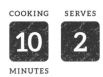

COOKING **10** MINUTES

SERVES **2**

1 teaspoon sesame seeds

1 x 120 g bag mixed salad leaves

3 baby cucumbers, sliced lengthways

2 French shallots, finely sliced

½ punnet (125 g) baby roma tomatoes, halved

½ small red onion, finely sliced

1 x 110 g tin pink salmon, drained

½ orange, peeled, segmented and deveined

2 tablespoons extra-virgin olive oil

Juice ½ lemon

Sea salt and freshly ground black pepper

CARAMELISED WALNUTS

2 tablespoons honey

12 walnut halves

This salad is rich in omega-3 fats and can be ready in minutes to enjoy after a long day.

Lightly toast the sesame seeds in a small frying pan over a medium heat, then set aside. Wipe the pan out with kitchen paper, then return it to the heat to make the caramelised walnuts. Add the honey to the pan and cook for a minute or two, then add the walnuts and gently toss to coat them in the honey. Once the honey starts to bubble, transfer the walnuts to a lightly oiled tray or board to cool and harden.

Put the salad leaves, cucumber, shallot, tomato and red onion in a serving bowl. Add the pink salmon and orange segments and gently toss everything together.

Dress the salad with the olive oil, lemon juice and salt and pepper, then scatter over the toasted sesame seeds and caramelised walnuts before serving.

NUTRITION COMPOSITION PER SERVE			
Nutrient	Average Qty per serving	%RDI F	M
Energy	2336 kj	28%	23%
Protein	29.7 g	41%	33%
Carbohydrate	37.3 g	15%	12%
Fat	31.2 g	39%	32%
Sodium	223 mg	11%	11%
Fibre	7.7 g	28%	20%

High in selenium and omega-3 fats and a good source of fibre

Radicchio with peach and buffalo mozzarella

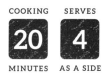

COOKING
20 MINUTES

SERVES
4 AS A SIDE

2 large white peaches (you can use yellow
   peaches if white aren't available),
   cut into segments

1 radicchio, leaves separated and
   roughly chopped

1 tablespoon extra-virgin olive oil

4 dates, pitted and finely sliced

1 tablespoon caramelised walnuts
   (see page 155)

1 large (150 g) burrata or large buffalo
   mozzarella

1 teaspoon balsamic glaze

1 teaspoon hazelnut meal or crushed
   pistachios

Ground nutmeg, to serve

Fresh herbs, if on hand

The bitterness of radicchio is nicely balanced by the sweetness
of peach and the richness of burrata or buffalo mozzarella.
An impressive salad to make for gatherings.

Preheat the oven to 200°C. Line a baking tray with baking paper
and roast the peaches for 20 minutes, or until softened and golden.
Set aside to cool completely.

Arrange the radicchio on a serving platter, drizzle over the olive
oil, carefully toss through the roasted peaches, dates and
caramelised walnuts.

Tear the burrata or buffalo mozzarella into five or six pieces and
arrange on the salad. Drizzle with the balsamic glaze and sprinkle
with the hazelnut meal or pistachios and a pinch of nutmeg, then
garnish with the fresh herbs, if on hand, before serving.

NUTRITION COMPOSITION PER SERVE			
Nutrient	Average Qty per serving	%RDI F	M
Energy	1126 kj	14%	11%
Protein	9.2 g	13%	10%
Carbohydrate	18.7 g	7%	6%
Fat	16.4 g	21%	17%
Sodium	65.9 mg	3%	3%
Fibre	4.7 g	17%	12%

High in calcium

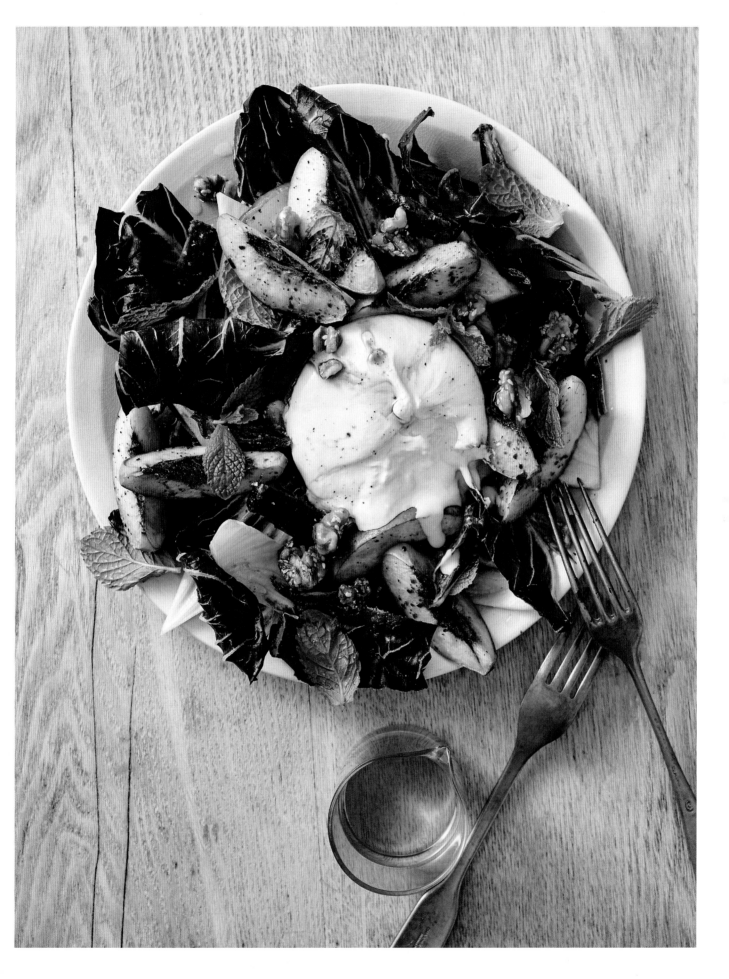

Leafy green salad with sugar snap peas and mustard dressing

100 g green beans, trimmed and cut into
5 cm lengths

100 g sugar snap peas

2 big handfuls mixed salad leaves

½ small red chilli, halved, deseeded
and finely sliced

10 pitted kalamata olives

2 plums, finely sliced

1 teaspoon pumpkin seeds, to serve

MUSTARD DRESSING

2 tablespoons extra-virgin olive oil

1 tablespoon wholegrain mustard

1 tablespoon lemon juice

Sea salt and freshly ground black pepper

The sugar snap peas add crunch to this leafy salad. They're called 'mangetout' in French, which literally means 'eat it all'.

Add all the dressing ingredients to a small jar and shake to combine.

Blanch the green beans and sugar snap peas in boiling water for a few minutes, or until bright green, then drain and allow to cool.

When ready to serve, put all the salad ingredients except the pumpkin seeds in a serving bowl, then drizzle over the dressing. Add the pumpkin seeds and gently toss everything together.

NUTRITION COMPOSITION PER SERVE			
Nutrient	Average Qty per serving	%RDI F	M
Energy	628 kj	8%	6%
Protein	2.7 g	4%	3%
Carbohydrate	5.4 g	2%	2%
Fat	12.3 g	15%	13%
Sodium	271 mg	14%	14%
Fibre	3.2 g	11%	8%

Wild leafy greens with garlic

COOKING
10
MINUTES

SERVES
4
AS A SIDE

4 cups (125 g) mixed wild greens or
cultivated varieties, such as chicory,
rocket, sorrel, endive or beetroot tops

2 tablespoons extra-virgin olive oil

Juice 1 lemon

2 garlic cloves, finely chopped

Sea salt and freshly ground black pepper

Wild edible greens, called horta in Greek, are a staple vegetable for foragers. These greens are rich in a group of antioxidants called carotenoids.

I recall collecting wild greens by the roadside in the outer suburbs of Melbourne with my family. A fairly common wild green is dandelion, which grows abundantly among wild grasses and even on lawns. Other varieties include wild or cultivated chicory, rocket, chard, sorrel or collards. Some with softer leaves, such as amaranth, only need a quick blanching; however, others such as wild chicory and dandelion are tougher and need at least 20 minutes of boiling.

Trim the wild greens, then wash thoroughly in plenty of water to remove any soil.

Place the greens in a large saucepan of boiling water and boil for 10 minutes, then remove from the heat, drain and place in a bowl.

Dress with the olive oil and lemon juice and add the garlic. Season lightly with salt and pepper (if you use plenty of lemon juice you will not need salt). Serve right away.

NUTRITION COMPOSITION PER SERVE			
Nutrient	Average Qty per serving	%RDI F	M
Energy	386 kj	5%	4%
Protein	0.7 g	1%	1%
Carbohydrate	0.7 g	0%	0%
Fat	9.4 g	12%	10%
Sodium	59 mg	3%	3%
Fibre	1.2 g	4%	3%

Black-eyed pea and vegetable soup

COOKING
40 MINUTES

SERVES
6

⅓ cup (80 ml) extra-virgin olive oil

1 leek, white and light green parts only, finely sliced and washed

1 celery stalk, finely sliced

1 small sweet potato, diced

1 small purple sweet potato, diced

1 small carrot, diced

¼ head of cauliflower, cut into florets

¼ head of broccoli, cut into florets

¾ cup (80 g) green beans, trimmed and cut into 5 cm lengths

1 zucchini, diced

200 g dried black-eyed peas, soaked overnight then par-cooked, or 1 x 400 g tin black-eyed peas, drained and rinsed (see note)

1 cup (250 ml) puréed tomato

1 x 400 g tin chopped tomatoes

4 cups (1 litre) boiling water

Sea salt and freshly ground black pepper

½ teaspoon ground turmeric

½ cup (25 g) baby spinach leaves

Fresh herbs, if on hand

A hearty Greek-style minestrone with black-eyed peas (also called cow peas), which are rich in protein, fibre and minerals, and spiced with turmeric, which has anti-inflammatory properties.

Heat 2 tablespoons of olive oil in a large pot over a medium heat and sauté the leek and celery for 5–10 minutes, or until starting to soften.

Add the rest of the vegetables – except the spinach – to the pot and continue to sauté until they are starting to soften. If using par-cooked black-eyed peas, add those now and stir through.

Add the tinned and puréed tomatoes and boiling water to the pot. Season with salt, pepper and turmeric, then simmer for 30 minutes, or until the vegetables are cooked through. If you are using tinned black-eyed peas, add these 10 minutes before the end of cooking.

Stir the baby spinach through the hot soup, drizzle over the rest of the olive oil and garnish with the fresh herbs, if on hand, just before serving.

TIP

Soaked dried black-eyed peas taste so much better than tinned. I like to soak 500 g or 1 kg of dried black-eyed peas overnight in water. The next day, I drain them, then divide them into smaller portions in zip-lock bags and freeze them so I have them ready to cook.

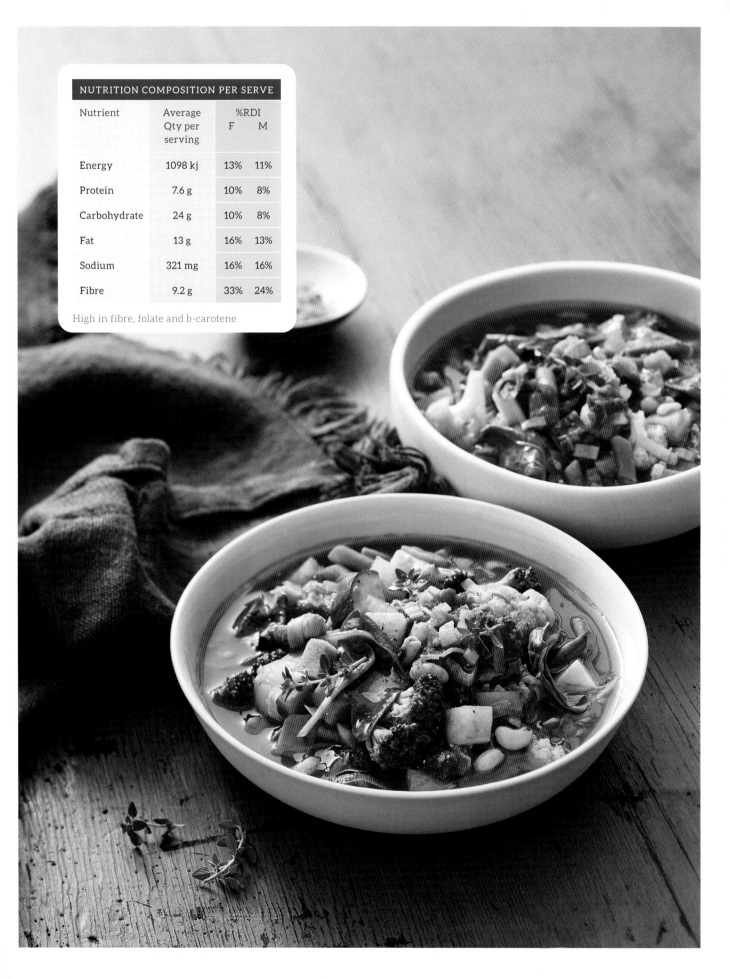

NUTRITION COMPOSITION PER SERVE

Nutrient	Average Qty per serving	%RDI F	M
Energy	1098 kj	13%	11%
Protein	7.6 g	10%	8%
Carbohydrate	24 g	10%	8%
Fat	13 g	16%	13%
Sodium	321 mg	16%	16%
Fibre	9.2 g	33%	24%

High in fibre, folate and b-carotene

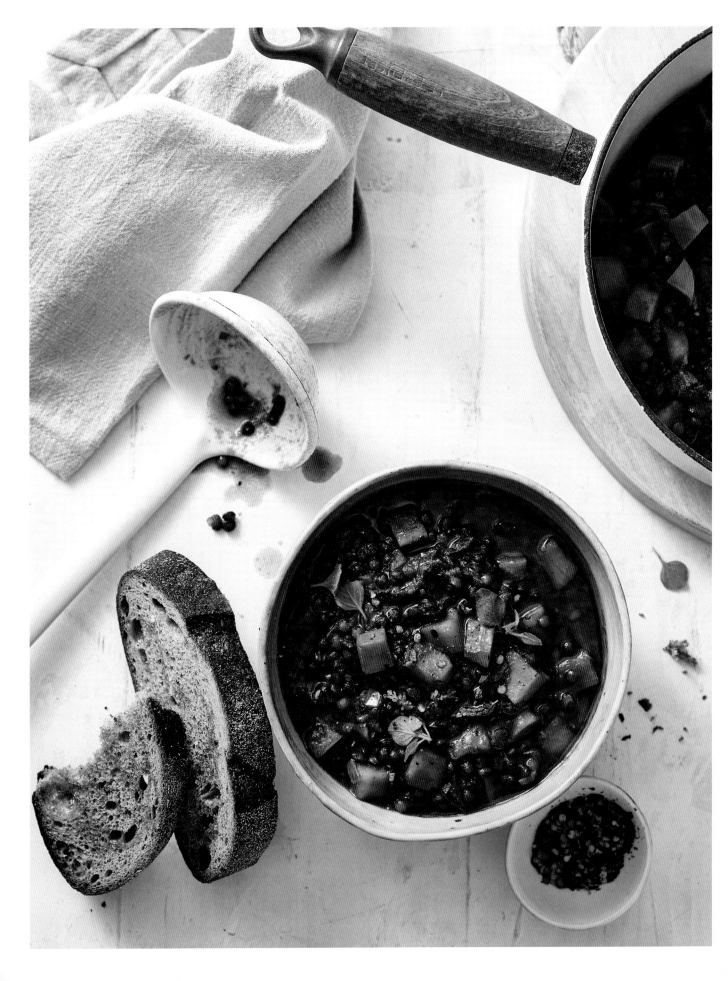

Spicy *lentil* and sweet potato soup

2 tablespoons extra-virgin olive oil

1 red onion, finely chopped

1 garlic clove, finely chopped

2 carrots, finely diced

1 white sweet potato, finely diced

1 small red chilli, finely sliced

¼ teaspoon ground nutmeg

375 g dried small brown lentils, rinsed

½ cup (125 ml) red wine

4 cups (1 litre) boiling water

½ cup (125 ml) puréed tomato

2 tomatoes, chopped

Sea salt and freshly ground black pepper

Optional: chilli flakes

1 tablespoon balsamic vinegar

Sourdough bread (see page 106), to serve

Fresh herbs, if on hand

Greek lentil soup (called fakes) was a favourite after-school snack for my daughters Tiana and Vivienne. This is a variation to suit their love for spicy foods, with sweet potato, chilli and aromatic spices to boost antioxidants. Keep leftovers refrigerated for lunch the next day, or freeze for a quick mid-week dinner.

Heat the olive oil in a large saucepan over a medium heat and sauté the onion and garlic until the onion is softened and translucent. Add the carrot, sweet potato, chilli and nutmeg and continue to sauté for around 10 minutes, or until the vegetables start to soften.

Add the lentils and red wine to the pan and simmer until most of the wine evaporates.

Next, add the water and puréed and chopped tomatoes to the pan and simmer for 30–45 minutes, or until the lentils and the sweet potato are cooked.

Season the soup with salt and pepper and add the chilli flakes if you like things spicy. Add a drizzle of balsamic vinegar, garnish with the fresh herbs, if on hand, then serve each portion with a slice of crusty sourdough.

NUTRITION COMPOSITION PER SERVE			
Nutrient	Average Qty per serving	%RDI F	M
Energy	1379 kj	17%	13%
Protein	16.6 g	23%	18%
Carbohydrate	40.9 g	16%	13%
Fat	7.6 g	10%	8%
Sodium	121 mg	6%	6%
Fibre	10.4 g	37%	27%

High in fibre

Healthy heart *minestrone*

⅓ cup (80 ml) extra-virgin olive oil

1 onion, finely diced

1 leek, white and light green parts,
   finely sliced and washed

1 fennel bulb, finely diced

3 celery stalks, finely diced

3 small carrots, finely diced

3 garlic cloves, finely diced

1 small red chilli, halved, deseeded
   and finely diced

½ teaspoon dried oregano

1 x 400 g tin chopped tomatoes

2 small zucchini, diced

10 g dried porcini mushrooms, soaked in
   boiling water for 10 minutes, drained
   and diced, soaking water reserved

1 x 400 g tin brown lentils, drained
   and rinsed

1 x 400 g tin chickpeas, drained and rinsed

1 x 400 g tin cannellini beans, drained
   and rinsed

8 cups (2 litres) low-salt vegetable stock

1 cup fresh casarecci (see note in intro),
   or dried red lentil pasta or green pea
   casarecci

½ bunch basil, leaves picked

60 g baby spinach leaves

Sea salt and freshly ground black pepper

Optional: finely grated parmesan, to serve

A hearty minestrone you could live on, this soup, created by my daughter Vivienne, includes a range of Mediterranean vegetables, fresh herbs, spices and three bean varieties to boost protein and fibre. This recipe makes a huge batch, so you can freeze in smaller portions if you wish.

Preferably use fresh pasta, or if using dried, cook separately and add towards the end, otherwise the soup will thicken too much.

Heat the olive oil in a large heavy-based saucepan over a medium–high heat and sauté the onion, leek, fennel, celery and carrot for 10–15 minutes, or until softened and lightly golden. Add the garlic, chilli, oregano, tomato, zucchini, porcini mushrooms, retained mushroom water from soaking, lentils, chickpeas, cannellini beans and vegetable stock. Stir and simmer for 30 minutes.

Add the pasta and cook according to packet instructions, or until al dente.

Tear the basil leaves into the soup and add the baby spinach. Season with salt and pepper to taste, and serve with a sprinkle of grated parmesan if you like.

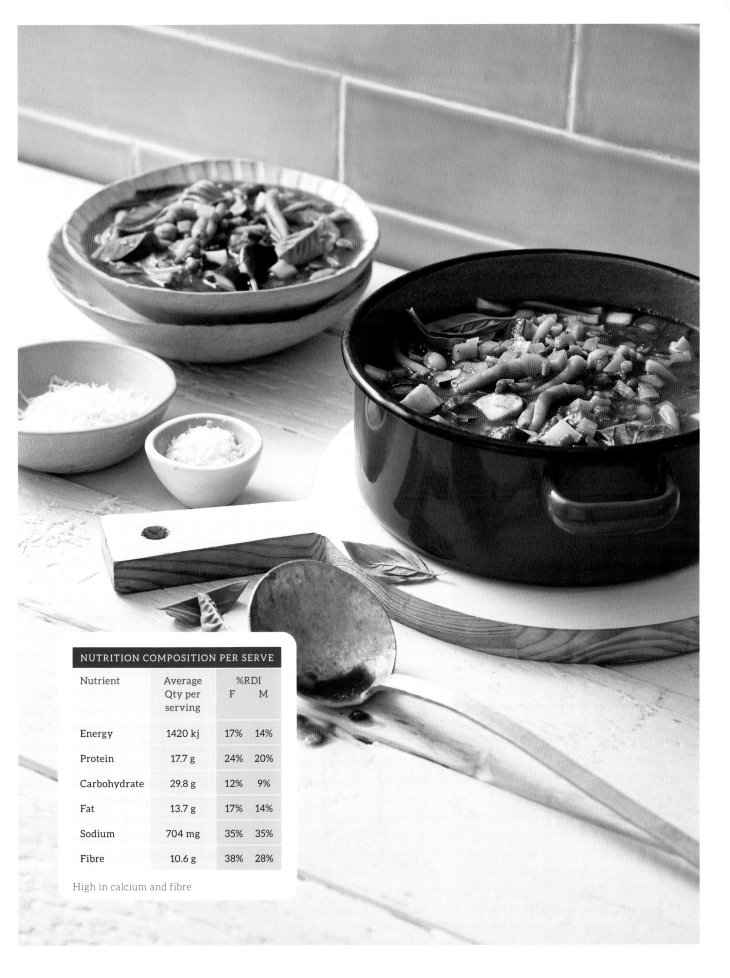

NUTRITION COMPOSITION PER SERVE			
Nutrient	Average Qty per serving	%RDI F	M
Energy	1420 kj	17%	14%
Protein	17.7 g	24%	20%
Carbohydrate	29.8 g	12%	9%
Fat	13.7 g	17%	14%
Sodium	704 mg	35%	35%
Fibre	10.6 g	38%	28%

High in calcium and fibre

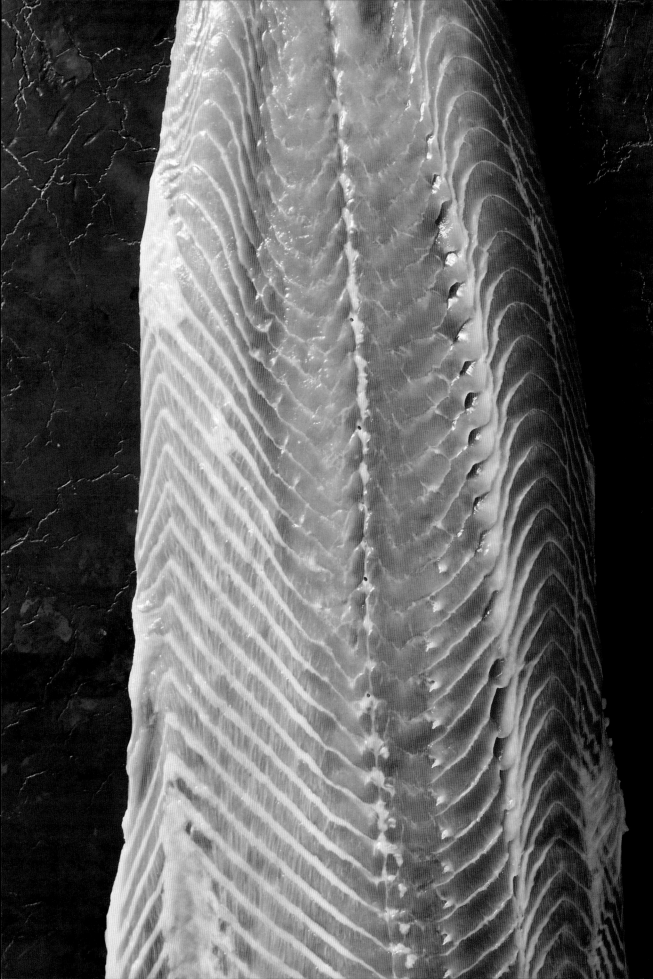

From the sea

—

Grilled *calamari* on cavolo nero pesto

2 tablespoons extra-virgin olive oil

300 g cleaned squid tubes (calamari), opened up, thickly sliced and scored, soaked in milk overnight in the fridge

1 garlic clove, crushed

Juice ½ lemon

Fresh herbs, if on hand

CAVOLO NERO PESTO

200 g cavolo nero (or kale, stalks removed), chopped and boiled until soft (3 minutes), drained

½ preserved lemon rind (see page 207), roughly chopped

⅓ cup (60 g) pine nuts

½ garlic clove, crushed

¼ cup (60 ml) extra-virgin olive oil

Sea salt and freshly ground black pepper

Squid is rich in protein, low in saturated fat and high in omega-3 fats, and commonly consumed fried and served with ouzo in Greece. In this dish the squid is grilled, which is a much healthier option.

Start by making the pesto. Place the boiled cavolo nero in a food processor with the chopped preserved lemon, pine nuts and garlic. Blitz until creamy, gradually adding the olive oil. Season with salt and pepper to taste.

Heat the olive oil in a chargrill pan over a medium heat. Once hot, chargrill the squid for a few minutes on both sides. Add the garlic – make sure it doesn't burn – then season with salt and pepper and squeeze over the lemon juice.

Spread the pesto on a serving plate and gently place the grilled calamari on top. Garnish with the fresh herbs, if on hand, and serve right away.

Nutrient	Average Qty per serving	%RDI F	M
Energy	1585 kj	19%	15%
Protein	15.4 g	21%	17%
Carbohydrate	1.5 g	1%	0%
Fat	34.5 g	43%	35%
Sodium	389 mg	19%	19%
Fibre	2.3 g	8%	6%

NUTRITION COMPOSITION PER SERVE

High in selenium and omega-3 fats

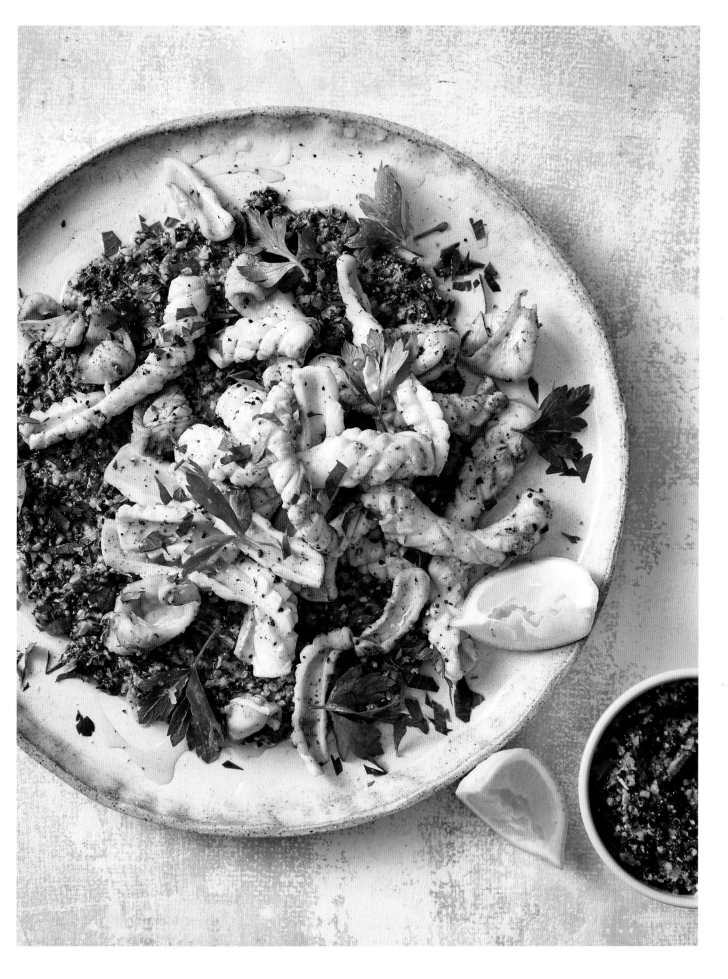

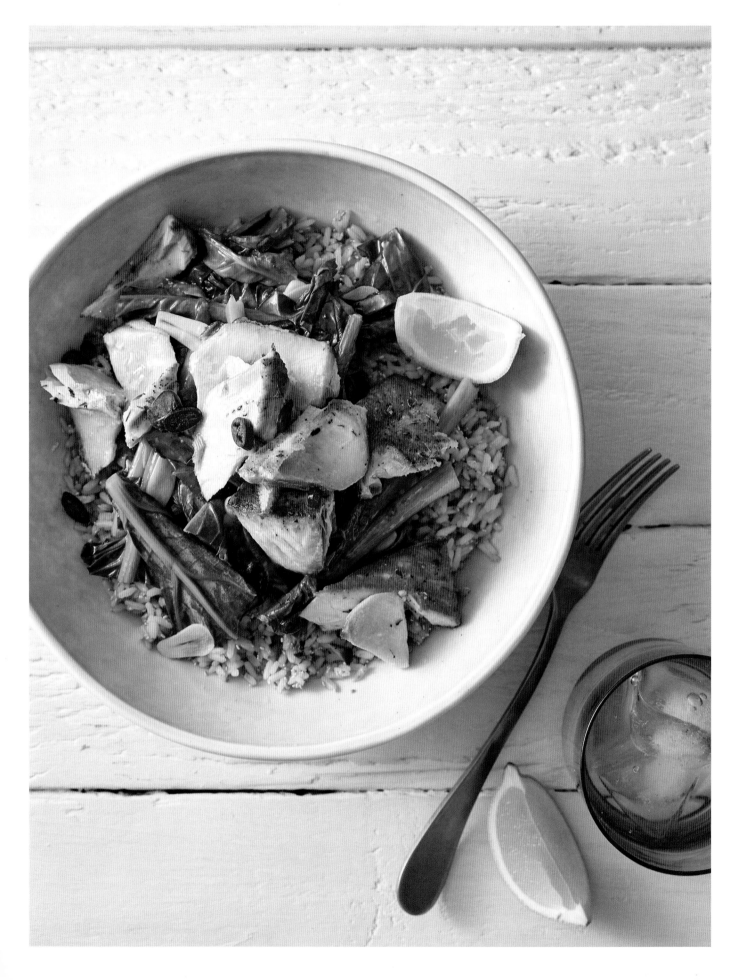

Salmon MediterrAsian Bowl

COOKING
15 MINUTES

SERVES
1

Dried thyme

Sea salt and freshly ground black pepper

1 x 180 g salmon fillet, skin on

2 tablespoons extra-virgin olive oil

2 garlic cloves, finely sliced

½ small red chilli, halved, deseeded
and finely sliced

½ bunch gai lan, bok choy or other Asian
green, trimmed and roughly chopped

2 teaspoons white wine vinegar

1 cup (250 g) microwaveable brown rice
and chia seeds

Lemon wedges, if on hand

This dish, rich in omega-3 fats, takes minutes to prepare and is ideal for a quick after-work meal or lunch on the run. You can cut corners by preparing wholemeal microwaveable rice while you quickly sear the fresh salmon and leafy greens.

Sprinkle a few pinches of dried thyme, salt and pepper over the salmon and rub in. Cut the salmon into 3 pieces.

Heat half the olive oil in a large heavy-based frying pan over a medium–high heat and sear the salmon for a few minutes on each side (or until cooked to your liking), then set aside in a bowl.

Return the pan to the heat, add the remaining olive oil and sauté the garlic and chilli for a few minutes (take care not to burn the garlic). Add the greens and sauté for a minute before adding the vinegar. Continue to cook for a few minutes, or until the greens are wilted. Add a splash of water to help the greens steam, then remove from the heat.

Transfer the greens to the bowl so they sit next to the salmon.

Quickly heat the brown rice and chia seeds according to the packet instructions, then add to a separate bowl. Top the rice with the wilted greens, then flake the salmon and place it on top of the greens. Garnish with the lemon wedges, if on hand, before serving.

NUTRITION COMPOSITION PER SERVE			
Nutrient	Average Qty per serving	%RDI F	M
Energy	3162 kj	38%	31%
Protein	38.7 g	53%	43%
Carbohydrate	43.8 g	18%	14%
Fat	45.4 g	57%	46%
Sodium	304 mg	15%	15%
Fibre	8.6 g	31%	23%

High in fibre, selenium and omega-3 fats

Tuna and vegetable
kebabs with pesto

COOKING **15** MINUTES

SERVES **4**

500 g tuna steaks, cut into cubes

8 baby zucchini, thickly sliced

1 red capsicum, deseeded and
  roughly diced

1 yellow capsicum, deseeded and
  roughly diced

4 red onions, quartered

8 bamboo skewers, soaked in water for
  20 minutes (or metal skewers)

Extra-virgin olive oil, for brushing

½ cup Traditional basil pesto
  (see page 84)

Fresh herbs and lemon wedges, if on hand

Salad or pilaf, to serve

A healthy omega-3-rich alternative to lamb kebabs. Perfect for parties and a fun way for children to enjoy fish.

Thread the tuna and vegetables onto the skewers with the onion alternating between the tuna and vegetables, and ensuring a piece of vegetable sits at either end of each skewer, to secure the kebab.

Place a chargrill pan over a medium heat and brush with the olive oil. Cook the kebabs until seared on all sides. The cooking time will vary depending on how you like your tuna and vegetables cooked, but ensure the fish is not overcooked as it will dry out too much.

Once cooked, place the kebabs on a serving dish. Garnish with the fresh herbs and lemon wedges, if on hand. Serve with the pesto for drizzling over the kebabs. This goes well with the Seychelles salad (see page 145), a simple tossed green salad or a side of Lentil pilaf (see page 116).

NUTRITION COMPOSITION PER SERVE*			
Nutrient	Average Qty per serving	%RDI F	M
Energy	1707 kj	21%	17%
Protein	37.6 g	52%	42%
Carbohydrate	17.3 g	7%	5%
Fat	19 g	24%	19%
Sodium	359 mg	18%	18%
Fibre	9 g	32%	24%

*Kebabs and basil pesto only
High in fibre and selenium,
moderate in omega-3 fats

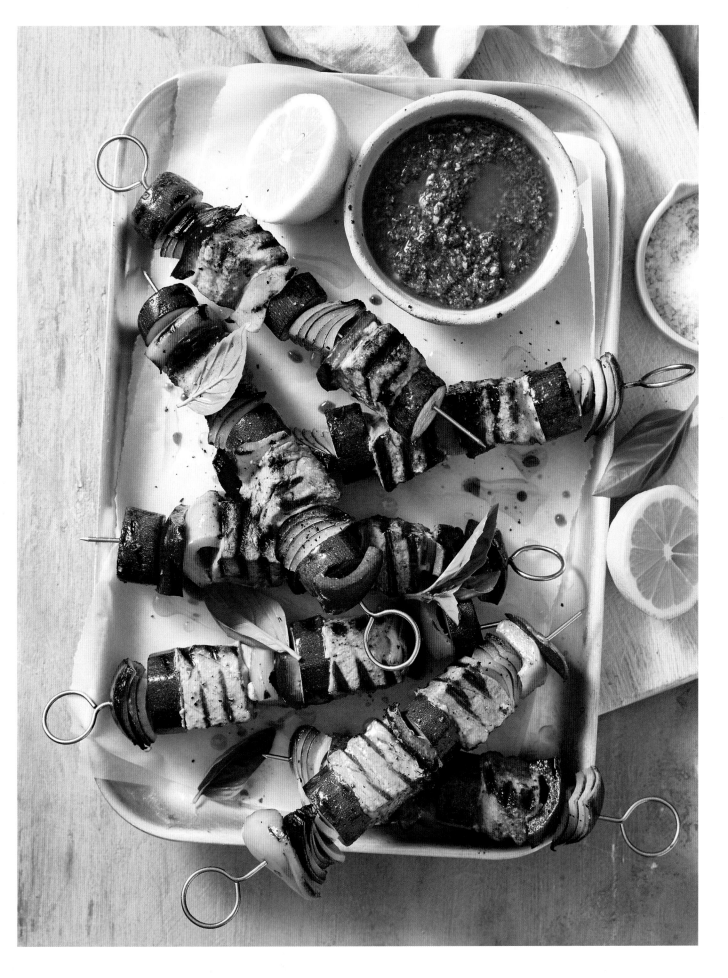

Easy *marinade* for tuna steaks and more

COOKING **10** MINUTES   SERVES **4**

4 x tuna steaks (about 1.5 cm thick)

1 tablespoon extra-virgin olive oil

1 red capsicum, deseeded and finely diced

Optional: 1 small red chilli, finely chopped

½ fennel bulb, finely chopped

Fresh herbs, if on hand

Salad, to serve

EASY MARINADE

½ teaspoon dried thyme

2 tablespoons extra-virgin olive oil

Juice ½ lemon, plus extra for serving

Sea salt and freshly ground black pepper

This is a great way to include one of your two serves of fish per week. Pick up tuna steaks from the supermarket on the way home, quickly chop up the fresh herbs and chilli while the tuna steaks are marinating, sear in a hot chargrill pan and serve with a tossed salad. Easy peasy.

Place the tuna steaks on a tray or in an airtight container. Mix the marinade ingredients in a large bowl, then spoon the marinade all over the tuna steaks to completely cover them. Cover and refrigerate for 1 hour.

When ready to cook, heat 1 tablespoon olive oil in a heavy-based frying pan or chargrill pan (or on a barbecue plate) over a medium–high heat and sear the tuna for 2–3 minutes on each side (or cook the tuna steaks to your taste but take care not to overcook them). Set aside.

Add the capsicum, chilli (if using) and fennel to the pan and cook for 2–3 minutes. Return the tuna to the pan. Garnish with the fresh herbs, if on hand, and squeeze over some extra lemon juice, then serve with a side salad of Charred cos lettuce with pangrattato and grated parmesan (see page 149).

NUTRITION COMPOSITION PER SERVE			
Nutrient	Average Qty per serving	%RDI F	M
Energy	1131 kj	14%	11%
Protein	34.8 g	48%	39%
Carbohydrate	5.2 g	2%	2%
Fat	10.9 g	14%	11%
Sodium	161 mg	8%	8%
Fibre	3.6 g	13%	9%

Moderate in omega-3 fats

Mussels with salsa verde and white wine

2 tablespoons extra-virgin olive oil

1 red onion, finely chopped

1 garlic clove, finely chopped

1 small red chilli, finely sliced

1 kg mussels, scrubbed and de-bearded

1 cup (250 ml) dry white wine

1 small handful of crushed pistachios
  or toasted pine nuts, to serve

4 thick slices sourdough bread (see
  page 106), to serve

SALSA VERDE

1 cup (60 g) flat-leaf parsley leaves, plus
  extra to serve

½ cup (30 g) mixed soft herbs such as dill,
  coriander and mint

½ cup (125 ml) extra-virgin olive oil

Mussels are a rich source of omega-3 fats and are inexpensive and low in kilojoules. What a great way to enjoy the Mediterranean diet.

Add all the salsa verde ingredients to a food processor, blend until puréed then set aside.

Heat the olive oil in a large pot over a medium heat and sauté the onion, garlic and chilli until the onion is softened and translucent.

Add the mussels to the pot, put on the lid and cook until the mussels pop open. Pour in the wine and cook for a few minutes more, until the alcohol cooks off, then add the salsa verde and toss well.

Garnish the mussels with the extra parsley and the crushed pistachios or toasted pine nuts. Serve with the sourdough right away.

NUTRITION COMPOSITION PER SERVE			
Nutrient	Average Qty per serving	%RDI F	M
Energy	2382 kj	29%	23%
Protein	46.6 g	64%	52%
Carbohydrate	12.4 g	5%	4%
Fat	35.4 g	44%	36%
Sodium	1082 mg	54%	54%
Fibre	2.8 g	10%	7%

High in omega-3 fats

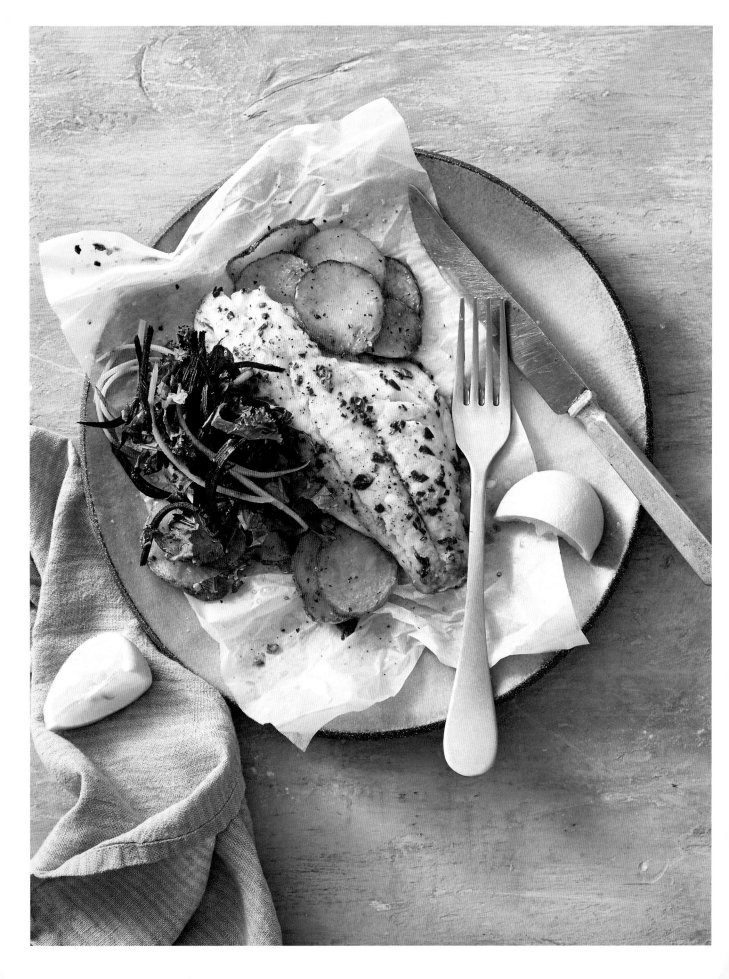

Fish parcel with beetroot slaw

1 x 120 g snapper fillet, skin and bones
removed (or other white fish)

Sea salt and freshly ground black pepper

1 tablespoon extra-virgin olive oil

¼ teaspoon fresh or dried thyme

½ garlic clove, finely chopped

¼ small red chilli, finely chopped

3 baby potatoes, sliced

½ cup beetroot slaw (pre-prepared,
from the supermarket)

Juice ½ lemon

Fresh herbs, if on hand

A healthy way to enjoy fish fillets is to cook them in foil or baking paper in the oven. This method can also minimise the fish smell in the house and reduce the cleaning of pots and pans.

Preheat the oven to 180°C. Line a baking tray with two large pieces of foil or baking paper, in a cross.

Season the snapper fillet with salt and pepper, then baste with half the olive oil and sprinkle over the thyme, garlic and chilli.

Heat the rest of the olive oil in a large frying pan over a medium heat and add the sliced potato and cook for 10 minutes, or until slightly golden on both sides. Transfer the potato to the middle of the foil or paper, then place the fish on top.

Fold the foil or paper over the fish to seal and make a parcel. Bake for 10 minutes. Meanwhile, dress the beetroot slaw with the lemon juice and season with salt and pepper to taste.

Remove the tray of fish from the oven, carefully open the parcel and garnish with the fresh herbs, if on hand, before serving with the beetroot slaw and an additional squeeze of lemon juice.

NUTRITION COMPOSITION PER SERVE			
Nutrient	Average Qty per serving	%RDI F	M
Energy	2160 kj	26%	21%
Protein	32.1 g	44%	36%
Carbohydrate	42.1 g	17%	13%
Fat	20.6 g	26%	21%
Sodium	321 mg	16%	16%
Fibre	8.4 g	30%	22%

High in fibre, selenium and iodine
and moderate in omega-3 fats

Quick *spaghetti* with salmon

COOKING **20** MINUTES

SERVES **2** OR 1 WITH LEFTOVERS

250 g gluten-free spaghetti

2 tablespoons extra-virgin olive oil,
plus extra for pasta

1 x 200 g salmon fillet, skin and bones
removed, cut into 2 cm pieces

1 red onion, finely diced

1 small red chilli, halved, deseeded
and finely sliced

1 garlic clove, finely diced

¼ cup (60 ml) dry white wine

½ punnet (125 g) baby roma tomatoes,
halved

1 small bunch broccolini, cut into
2 cm pieces

Sea salt and freshly ground black pepper

Lemon wedges, if on hand

This pasta dish of seared salmon, tomatoes and herbs is ideal for a quick after-work meal. Just add a glass of chilled wine.

Place a large saucepan of salted water on to boil. Add the spaghetti and a few drops of olive oil, and cook according to packet instructions, or until al dente.

Meanwhile, heat the olive oil in a large frying pan over a medium heat. Add the salmon and cook for 2–3 minutes on each side. Transfer to a plate and cover to keep warm.

Add the onion to the pan and sauté until softened and translucent. Add the chilli and garlic and continue to cook (taking care not to burn the garlic). Pour in the wine, and swirl it around the pan to deglaze. Allow most of the alcohol to evaporate before adding the tomato and broccolini. Cook the vegetables for a few minutes. Break the salmon into pieces and gently toss through.

When the pasta is cooked, drain it and add to the pan with the salmon and vegetables. Toss everything together gently, season with salt and pepper to taste and garnish with the lemon wedges, if on hand, just before serving.

NUTRITION COMPOSITION PER SERVE			
Nutrient	Average Qty per serving	%RDI F	M
Energy	3721 kj	45%	36%
Protein	39.8 g	55%	44%
Carbohydrate	91.7 g	37%	29%
Fat	37.5 g	47%	38%
Sodium	140 mg	7%	7%
Fibre	8.6 g	31%	23%

High in omega-3 fats and a good source of fibre

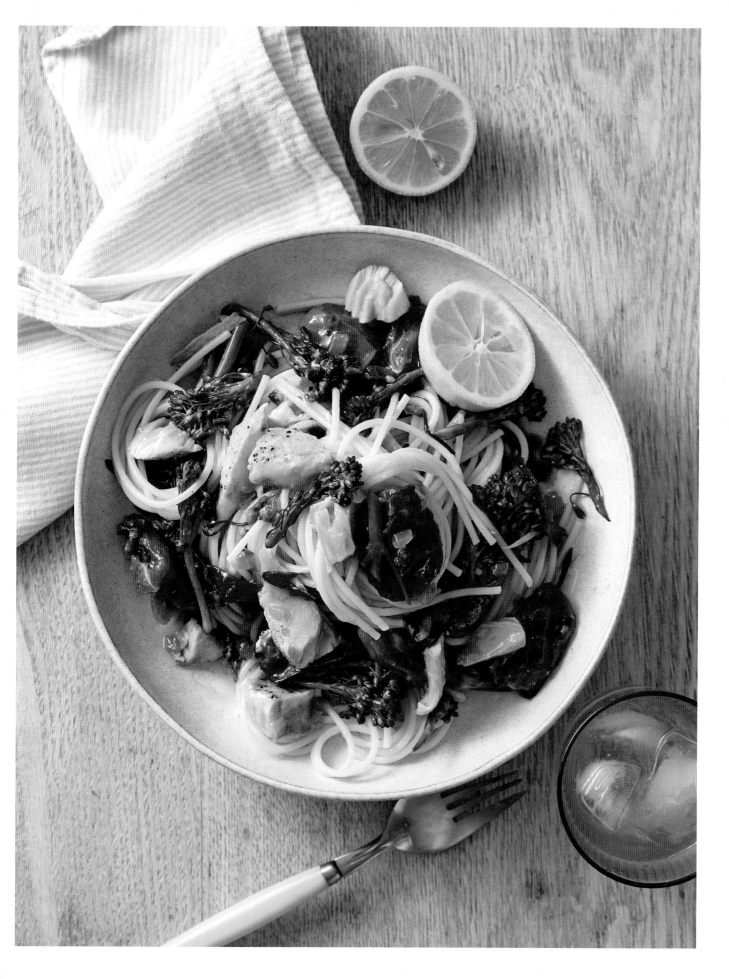

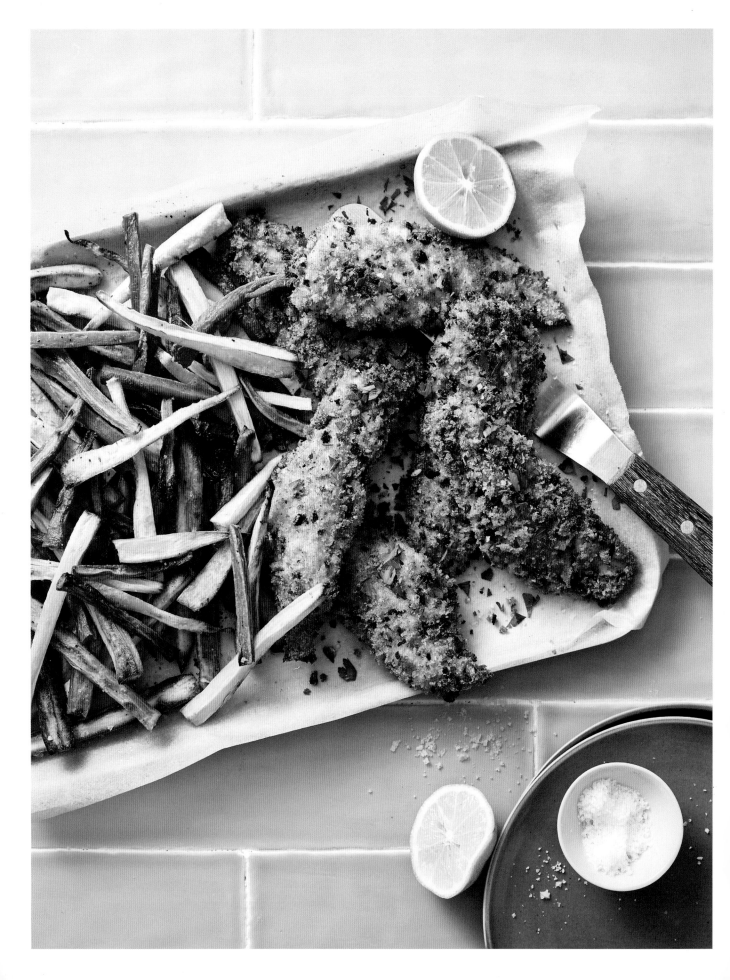

Healthy *fish and chips*

COOKING **30** MINUTES

SERVES **4**

500 g flathead or other white fish fillets,
  such as snapper, blue-eye trevalla or
  whiting, skin and bones removed

2 eggs, lightly beaten

½ cup (50 g) wholegrain breadcrumbs
  (or gluten-free if preferred)

1 sweet potato, cut into chips

1 purple sweet potato, cut into chips

2 parsnips, cut into chips

2 large carrots, cut into chips

Extra-virgin olive oil, for brushing

Sea salt and freshly ground black pepper

Fresh herbs and lemon wedges, if on hand

Following a heart healthy diet does not mean you need to miss out on fish and chips! Try different fillets and be adventurous with the vegetable chips for colour and variety.

Line two large baking trays with baking paper. Dip each fish fillet in the beaten egg, coating completely. Let any excess drip off, then dip in the breadcrumbs to coat completely. Place on one prepared tray, cover, then refrigerate for 1 hour.

Preheat the oven to 200°C. Spread the vegetables around the other prepared tray and brush with the olive oil. Season generously with salt and pepper and roast for 30 minutes, turning halfway through if needed, until golden and crisp.

Meanwhile, transfer the fish to the oven to bake for 15–20 minutes, or until it is golden and cooked through. Garnish with the fresh herbs and lemon wedges, if on hand, and serve.

NUTRITION COMPOSITION PER SERVE			
Nutrient	Average Qty per serving	%RDI F	M
Energy	1762 kj	21%	17%
Protein	33.9 g	46%	38%
Carbohydrate	36.7 g	15%	11%
Fat	13.2 g	17%	13%
Sodium	405 mg	20%	20%
Fibre	8.4 g	30%	22%

Good source of fibre

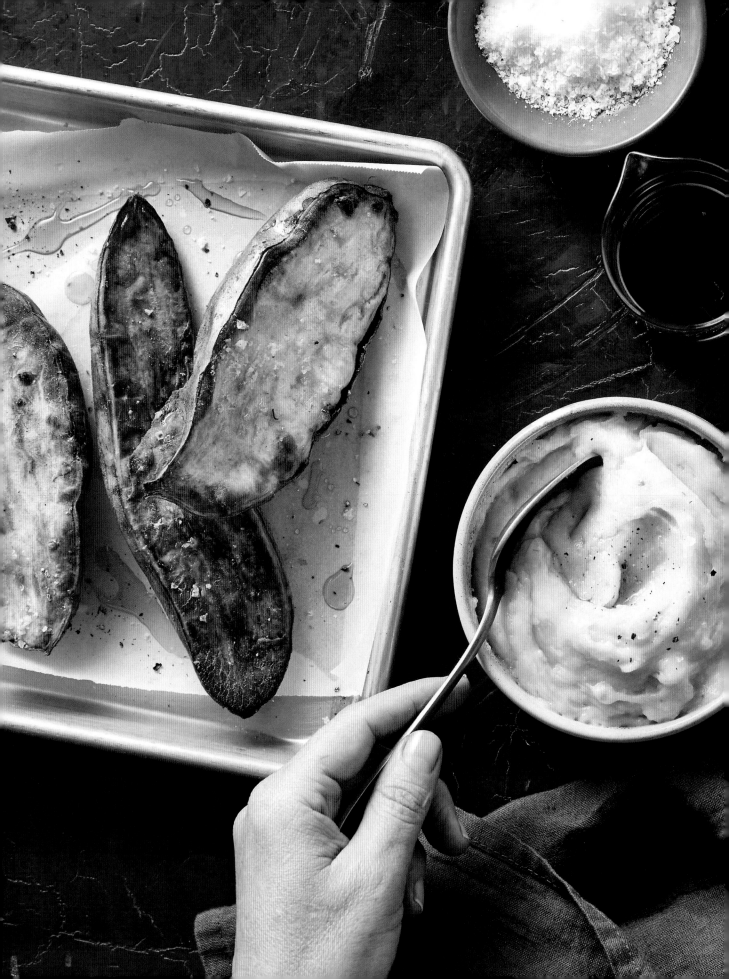

Skordalia: purple-skinned white sweet potato and garlic mash

COOKING
20
MINUTES

SERVES
4

1 large purple-skinned white sweet potato (about 500 g), peeled and roughly chopped

⅓ cup (80 ml) extra-virgin olive oil, plus extra for roasting

½ teaspoon sea salt, plus extra for seasoning

2 garlic gloves, finely chopped

⅓ cup (80 ml) lemon juice

Freshly ground black pepper

This is a variation on the Greek potato dish skordalia, which goes perfectly well with fish, meatballs or baked vegetables (especially beetroot). Sweet potato has a lower GI than potato and is better for people with diabetes. You can boil the sweet potatoes rather than roast them, but roasting will give the skordalia a richer flavour and creamier texture.

Preheat the oven to 200°C. Line a baking tray with baking paper and spread the chunks of sweet potato out around the tray. Drizzle lightly with olive oil and add the salt, then roast for 15–20 minutes, or until soft. Remove from the oven, and cover to keep warm.

Using a hand-held blender or food processor, blend the olive oil, garlic and lemon juice until they form a smooth purée.

Mash the warm sweet potato using a drum sieve, mouli grater or food mill (you may need to repeat this step to get a really smooth mash). This can also be done in a food processor.

Add the olive oil mixture to the mash and stir until thick and smooth. Taste to check seasoning, then serve with a main meal – it's perfect with fish and wilted wild greens.

NUTRITION COMPOSITION PER SERVE

Nutrient	Average Qty per serving	%RDI F	M
Energy	470 kj	6%	5%
Protein	0.6 g	1%	1%
Carbohydrate	9.9 g	4%	3%
Fat	7.5 g	9%	8%
Sodium	120 mg	6%	6%
Fibre	1.5 g	5%	4%

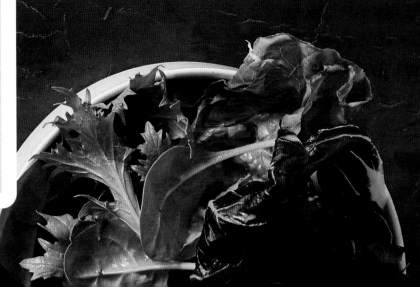

Marinated *white anchovies* with kritamos

SERVES

4

AS A
STARTER

1½ cups (250 g) pickled kritamos
  (see note)

1 small red onion, finely sliced

½ punnet (125 g) baby roma tomatoes,
  halved or quartered

250 g jar marinated white anchovies

Extra-virgin olive oil

Juice 1 lemon

Sea salt and freshly ground black pepper

Fresh herbs, if on hand

4 thick slices sourdough bread (see
  page 106), toasted, to serve

Kritamos is a wild succulent plant that grows along the Mediterranean coast. It is also called sea fennel and is popular in Cretan cuisine. It is pickled like capers and used in salads and tastes like a mixture of fennel and peppermint. It is rich in antioxidant minerals.

Gently toss the kritamos with the onion and tomato and place on a serving plate. Place the marinated white anchovies on top, then dress with olive oil, lemon juice and season with salt and pepper to taste (keeping in mind that the anchovies will be salty).

Garnish with the fresh herbs, if on hand, and serve with the toasted sourdough bread.

NOTE

Pickled kritamos is rock samphire or sea fennel, and it can be found in Mediterranean delicatessens. It can be substituted with sautéed wild greens such as dandelion, stinging nettles or wild chicory.

NUTRITION COMPOSITION PER SERVE			
Nutrient	Average Qty per serving	%RDI F	M
Energy	1032 kj	13%	10%
Protein	21.8 g	30%	24%
Carbohydrate	2.5 g	1%	1%
Fat	15.3 g	19%	16%
Sodium	3500 mg	175%	175%
Fibre	5.4 g	19%	14%

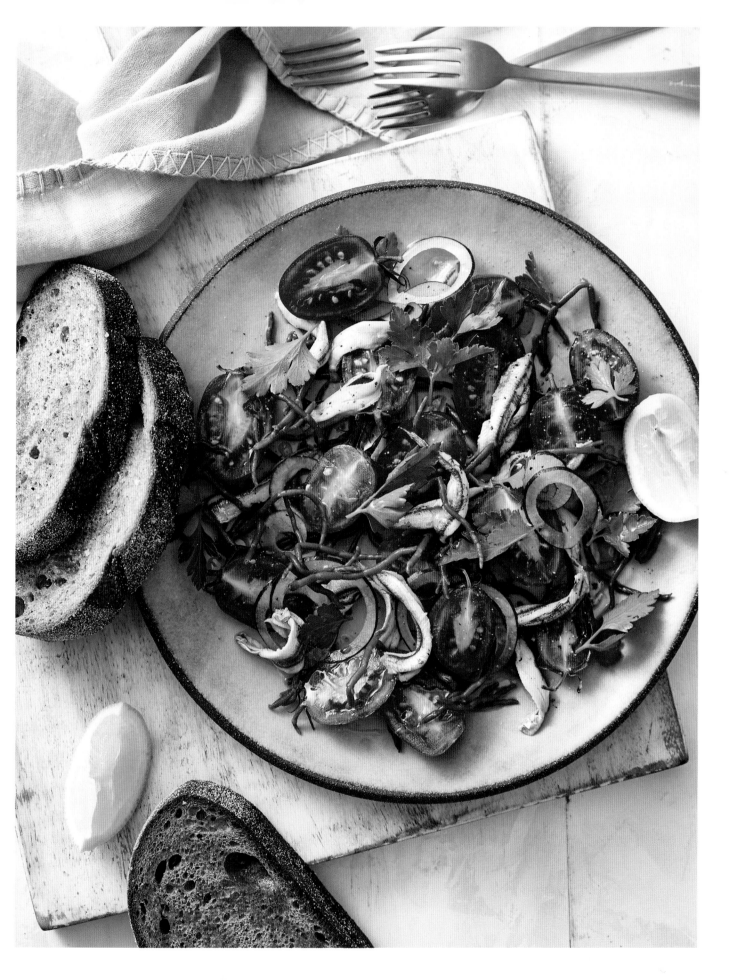

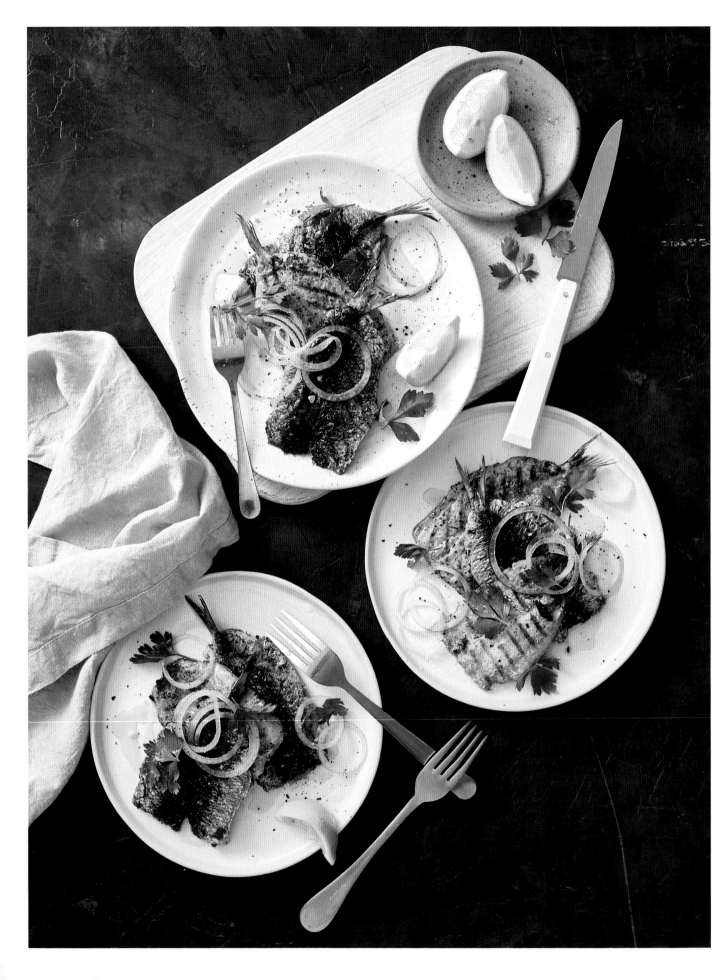

Chargrilled *sardine fillets*

COOKING
6
MINUTES

SERVES
4

16–20 (about 500 g) fresh sardines
 (or 12 pilchards)

1 teaspoon thyme leaves

Sea salt and freshly ground black pepper

Extra-virgin olive oil, for grilling

1 small red onion, finely sliced

Juice ½ lemon

Flat-leaf parsley leaves, if on hand

Salad and sautéed wild greens, to serve

Sardines are the richest source of omega-3 fats in the Mediterranean cuisine. Chargrilled and dressed with extra-virgin olive oil and lemon is a delicious way to enjoy these small fish. This dish is a showstopper at parties.

Scale the sardines, then remove their intestines, heads and tails. Wash them well, then open them out, butterfly-style (if you prefer, you can ask a fishmonger to do these things for you).

Sprinkle the thyme leaves over the sardines, add some salt and pepper, then drizzle with a little olive oil.

Heat a chargrill pan over a medium heat and drizzle on some olive oil. Add the sardines and chargrill for a few minutes on each side, then remove to a serving platter. Garnish with the sliced onion, a squeeze of lemon juice and a sprinkle of parsley, if on hand.

Serve with Fresh tomato salad (see page 141) and Sautéed wild greens (see page 89).

NUTRITION COMPOSITION PER SERVE			
Nutrient	Average Qty per serving	%RDI F	M
Energy	956 kj	12%	9%
Protein	25.4 g	35%	28%
Carbohydrate	1.7 g	1%	1%
Fat	1.5 g	2%	2%
Sodium	911 mg	46%	46%
Fibre	1.5 g	5%	4%

Very high in calcium and high in selenium, iodine and omega-3 fats

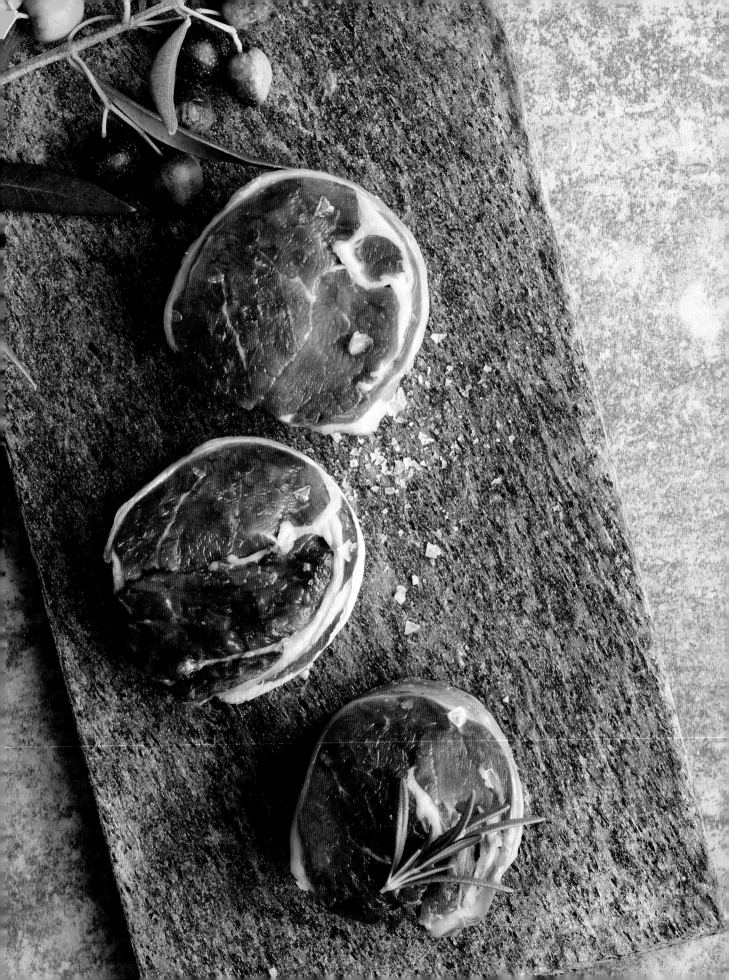

From the pasture

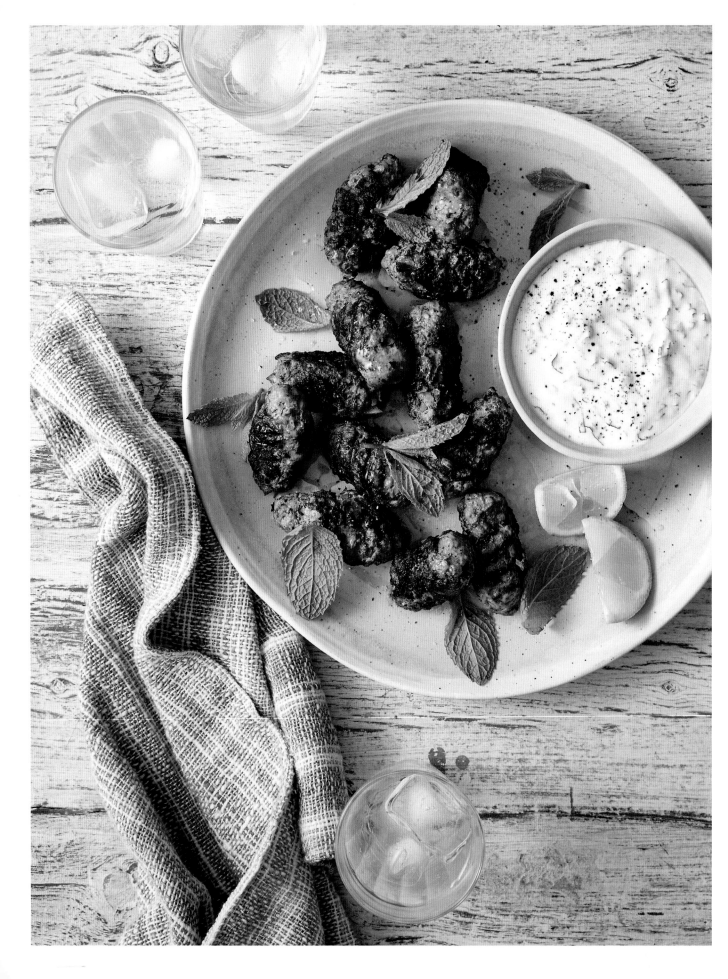

Souzoukakia

15 MINUTES

SERVES
6

500 g lean minced lamb

1 large onion, finely chopped

1 garlic clove, finely chopped

1 tomato, grated (see tip on page 97)

2–3 dill fronds, chopped

1 teaspoon dried oregano

1 small red chilli, finely chopped, or
   ½ teaspoon chilli flakes

¼ cup (60 ml) ouzo (anise-flavoured liquor)

1 tablespoon extra-virgin olive oil, plus
   extra for cooking

Sea salt and freshly ground black pepper

1 egg, lightly beaten

2 tablespoons wholemeal breadcrumbs
   (or rice crumbs for a gluten-free option)

Herb yoghurt (see page 205), to serve

Fresh herbs and lemon wedges, if on hand

These spicy finger-shaped patties (Greek-style chevaps) have a kick of ouzo and a Middle-Eastern influence that makes them perfect for mezedes with pre-dinner drinks. They can be enjoyed hot or cold and are best served with the Herb yoghurt on page 205 and Greco–Italian salad on page 196. This dish is also very easy to cook on a barbecue when the weather is nice.

Line a large baking tray with baking paper. Place the lamb mince in a large bowl and add the onion, garlic, tomato, dill, oregano, chilli, ouzo, olive oil and a good pinch of salt and pepper. Mix together well using clean hands.

Add the egg and breadcrumbs to the lamb mince mixture and mix until incorporated. With lightly oiled hands, roll small portions of the mixture into finger-shaped patties, then arrange these on the tray. Cover and refrigerate for 30 minutes to 1 hour.

When ready to cook the chevaps, drizzle a little olive oil onto a hot grill plate over a medium–high heat and chargrill the chevaps for 5–10 minutes, or until browned on all sides. Break open the first one you grill, to check that it's cooked through; make sure the outside colour is good and that the juices inside run clear.

Serve the chevaps with the Herb yoghurt and the fresh herbs and lemon wedges, if on hand.

NUTRITION COMPOSITION PER SERVE			
Nutrient	Average Qty per serving	%RDI F	M
Energy	947 kj	11%	9%
Protein	21 g	29%	23%
Carbohydrate	4.6 g	2%	1%
Fat	11.2 g	14%	11%
Sodium	149 mg	7%	7%
Fibre	1.4 g	5%	4%

FROM THE PASTURE   191

Kangaroo meatballs and spaghetti

300 g kangaroo mince or other lean
  mince such as veal

1 red onion, finely chopped

1 garlic clove, finely chopped

1 tomato, grated (see tip on page 97)

2–3 coriander sprigs, finely chopped

2–3 flat-leaf parsley sprigs, finely chopped

Optional: 1 small green chilli, halved,
  deseeded and finely chopped

1 teaspoon finely grated ginger

1 tablespoon extra-virgin olive oil,
  plus extra

Sea salt and freshly ground black pepper

1 egg

3 tablespoons gluten-free breadcrumbs

500 g wholemeal spaghetti (or gluten-free
  if preferred)

Optional: finely grated parmesan cheese,
  to serve

SAUCE

2 tablespoons extra-virgin olive oil

1 small red onion, finely chopped

1 garlic clove, finely chopped

1 cup (250 ml) puréed tomato

1 cup (250 ml) boiling water

1 fresh bay leaf

This dish is a variation on the traditional Italian spaghetti and meatballs, but uses kangaroo mince for that Australian-Mediterranean twist. Kangaroo is a very lean meat, rich in iron and low in saturated fats. It's a great way to enjoy meat dishes using local free-range produce.

Line a baking tray with baking paper. Place the mince in a bowl with the onion, garlic, tomato, herbs, chilli (if using), ginger, olive oil and salt and pepper. Mix well using clean hands. Add the egg and breadcrumbs and mix again until well combined.

Using lightly oiled hands, roll small portions of the mixture into walnut-sized balls. place on the baking tray, cover and refrigerate for 30 minutes to 1 hour.

When ready to cook, heat some extra olive oil in a large frying pan over a medium heat. Once hot, gently place the meatballs in the pan and fry until lightly golden on all sides. The meatballs can be partly cooked through as they will continue to cook in the sauce. Once golden, remove and place on a plate covered with kitchen paper to drain any excess oil.

To make the sauce, place a large saucepan over a medium heat and add the olive oil. Sauté the onion for a few minutes, then add the garlic, tomato, water and bay leaf. Season with salt and pepper. Simmer for 5 minutes until piping hot. Add the meatballs to the pan and continue to simmer for 10 minutes. Add a little extra boiling water if the sauce appears too thick.

Bring a large saucepan of water to the boil, add salt and a few drops of olive oil. Cook the spaghetti according to packet instructions, or until al dente, then drain.

Serve bowls of spaghetti with the meatballs and sauce on top. Sprinkle with the parmesan, if desired.

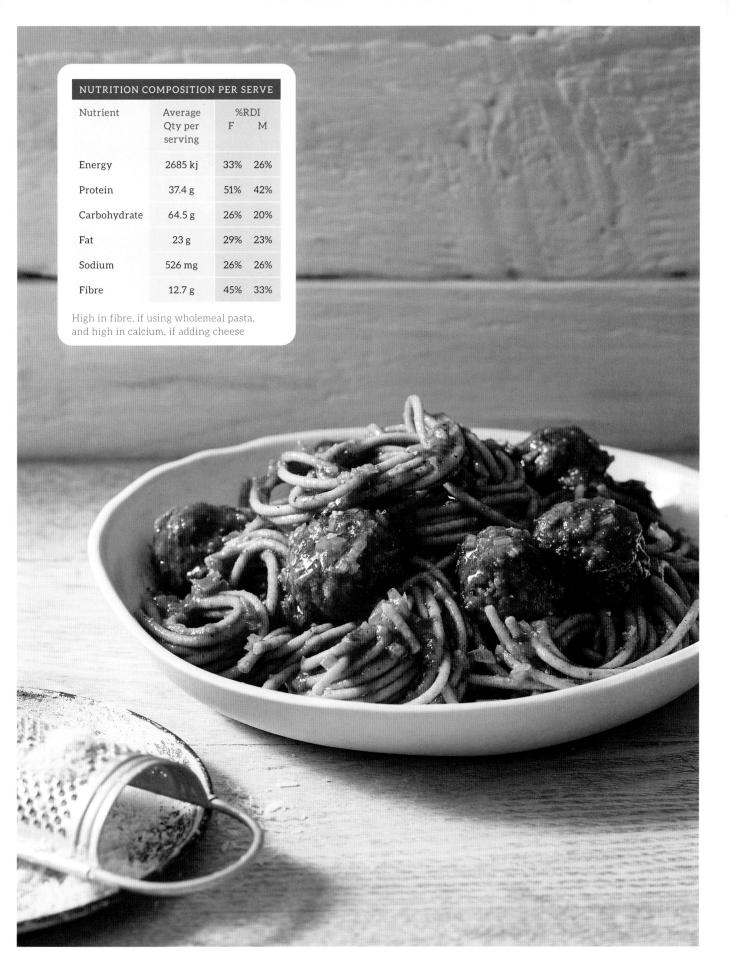

NUTRITION COMPOSITION PER SERVE

Nutrient	Average Qty per serving	%RDI F	M
Energy	2685 kj	33%	26%
Protein	37.4 g	51%	42%
Carbohydrate	64.5 g	26%	20%
Fat	23 g	29%	23%
Sodium	526 mg	26%	26%
Fibre	12.7 g	45%	33%

High in fibre, if using wholemeal pasta,
and high in calcium, if adding cheese

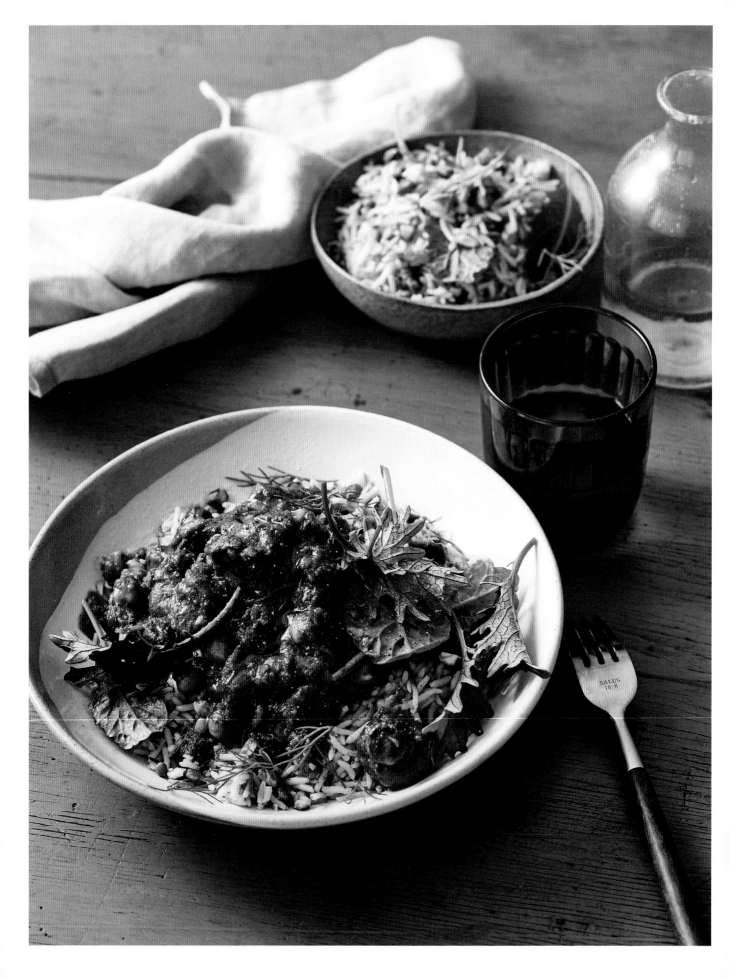

Spicy *slow-cooked lamb* with chickpeas

COOKING
2
HOURS +
20 MINUTES

SERVES
6

¼ cup (60 ml) extra-virgin olive oil

1 onion, diced

500 g lamb shoulder, diced

½ cup (125 ml) red wine

250 g French shallots, peeled

250 g button mushrooms, cleaned

½ teaspoon black peppercorns

1 fresh bay leaf

¼ teaspoon ground cumin

¼ teaspoon chilli powder

¼ teaspoon smoked paprika

1 teaspoon mixed dried herbs

2 cups (500 ml) puréed tomato

4 cups (1 litre) boiling water

2 x 400 g tins chickpeas, drained
    and rinsed

Sea salt and freshly ground black pepper

Lentil pilaf (see page 116), to serve

A hearty lamb casserole with Eastern Mediterranean spices to boost flavour and antioxidants, and enriched with chickpeas for fibre. Try serving this with the Lentil pilaf on page 116.

Heat the olive oil in a large saucepan over a medium heat and sauté the onion until softened and translucent. Add the lamb and sear on all sides, then deglaze the pan with the red wine. Cook for a few minutes to allow the alcohol to evaporate, add the shallots and mushrooms and allow to brown. Add the peppercorns, bay leaf, cumin, chilli powder, paprika and dried herbs.

Pour in the puréed tomato and half the boiling water, then reduce the heat to low and simmer the casserole for 1 ½ hours.

Remove a piece of lamb from the pan and check it. If it's still tough, add another 2 cups (500 ml) of boiling water and continue to simmer for another 20–30 minutes. Add the chickpeas and simmer for 10 minutes, then season with salt and pepper to taste and serve with Lentil pilaf, if desired.

NUTRITION COMPOSITION PER SERVE			
Nutrient	Average Qty per serving	%RDI F	M
Energy	1633 kj	20%	16%
Protein	31.7 g	43%	35%
Carbohydrate	18.5 g	7%	6%
Fat	18.1 g	23%	18%
Sodium	508 mg	25%	25%
Fibre	8.8 g	31%	23%

Spicy *lamb ribs*

1 kg lamb ribs

2 tablespoons extra-virgin olive oil

½ teaspoon ground cumin

¼ teaspoon chilli powder

½ teaspoon chilli flakes

1 teaspoon dried thyme

1 tablespoon finely chopped rosemary

½ teaspoon freshly ground black pepper

Sea salt

Herb yoghurt (see page 205), to serve

GRECO-ITALIAN SALAD

1 tablespoon pine nuts, toasted

4 handfuls mixed green salad leaves

4 roma tomatoes, diced

1 red onion, finely sliced

4 baby red capsicums, sliced

2 Lebanese cucumbers, diced

12 Sicilian green olives, pitted and sliced

Handful basil leaves

Optional: 1 tablespoon grated mizithra
cheese or parmesan and 1 thick slice
sourdough bread (see page 106), diced

DRESSING

2 tablespoons extra-virgin olive oil,
plus extra for croutons

1 tablespoon red wine vinegar

1 teaspoon mixed dried herbs

This traditional lamb dish, cooked on charcoal or in the oven for ease, is perfect as finger food for parties. It goes well with the Fresh tomato salad (see page 141) or this Greco-Italian salad, which is the perfect choice when you can't decide if you want a Greek or Italian salad.

Preheat the oven to 150°C. Line a baking tray with baking paper. Place the lamb ribs on the prepared tray and rub with the olive oil. Rub the herbs, spices and a few pinches of salt all over the ribs so they are well covered. Cover the tray with foil and roast for 2 hours.

Remove the foil from the tray, turn the oven temperature up to 200°C, then return the ribs to the oven to brown for 10 minutes.

Place all the salad ingredients except the cheese and croutons in a large serving bowl. Put all the dressing ingredients in a jar and shake to combine, then season with salt and pepper to taste. Drizzle the dressing over the salad then gently toss everything together and sprinkle the cheese and croutons on top (if using).

If you want crispy croutons for your salad, reduce the oven temperature to 180°C and spread the bread cubes around a baking tray. Drizzle well with olive oil and toss gently to coat them completely, then toast for 10 minutes, or until golden. Allow to cool before adding to the salad.

Serve the ribs with the Greco-Italian salad and Herb yoghurt.

NUTRITION COMPOSITION PER SERVE			
Nutrient	Average Qty per serving	%RDI F	M
Energy	2648 kj	32%	26%
Protein	43 g	59%	48%
Carbohydrate	4.5 g	2%	1%
Fat	49.3 g	62%	50%
Sodium	371 mg	19%	19%
Fibre	2.2 g	8%	6%

Capsicums stuffed with kangaroo mince and brown rice

1 tablespoon extra-virgin olive oil, plus extra ¼ cup (60 ml) for baking

1 red onion, finely chopped

1 garlic clove, finely chopped

300 g kangaroo mince

½ cup (100 g) long-grain brown or wild rice

Optional: ½ cup (125 ml) dry white wine

2 tomatoes, grated (see tip on page 97) or 1 cup (250 ml) puréed tomato

2 cups (500 ml) boiling water, plus extra ½ cup (125 ml) for baking

2–3 thyme sprigs, chopped

2–3 flat-leaf parsley sprigs, chopped

Sea salt and freshly ground black pepper

6 small round capsicums, tops cut off and reserved, seeds removed

Mixed leaf green salad, to serve

Feta, diced, to serve

A traditional Greek Mediterranean dish with a difference. Here I have used kangaroo in place of lamb or beef mince to give the dish an Australiana touch. Kangaroo is a local wild meat rich in iron and low in saturated fat.

Heat a drizzle of olive oil in a large heavy-based saucepan over a medium heat and sauté the onion until softened and translucent. Add the garlic and continue to sauté for a few minutes. Add the mince and fry until the meat is browned, breaking it up with a spoon as it cooks.

Add the rice to the pan, stir in the wine (if using) and cook for a few minutes until most of the alcohol evaporates. Then add the tomato and 2 cups of boiling water and simmer for about 10 minutes, or until the rice softens. If the rice is still crunchy after this time, add another cup of boiling water and cook until most of it is absorbed.

Add the herbs and season with salt and pepper to taste. Let the mixture cool for 10–15 minutes.

Preheat the oven to 180°C. Stand the capsicums in a baking dish, tops facing up, and carefully spoon the meat mixture into each cavity, filling to the top. Put the reserved capsicum lids back on.

Pour ¼ cup (60 ml) of olive oil and ½ cup (125 ml) of boiling water around the capsicums in the dish, then bake for 45 minutes, checking regularly so that the capsicums don't burn. Add another splash of boiling water if the dish is dry.

Once the rice filling is cooked, allow the capsicums to cool and serve with a mixed green salad and cubes of feta.

NUTRITION COMPOSITION PER SERVE			
Nutrient	Average Qty per serving	%RDI F	M
Energy	1119 kj	14%	11%
Protein	18.1 g	25%	20%
Carbohydrate	20.6 g	8%	6%
Fat	10.1 g	13%	10%
Sodium	35.5 mg	2%	2%
Fibre	7.9 g	28%	21%

Turkey meatballs
on creamy polenta

COOKING
35
MINUTES

SERVES
4

MEATBALLS

300 g turkey (or chicken) mince

2 tablespoons extra-virgin olive oil,
  plus extra for frying

1 onion, finely chopped

1 tomato, grated (see tip on page 97)

2 tablespoons gluten-free breadcrumbs

1 garlic clove, finely chopped

1 tablespoon finely grated ginger

2–3 coriander sprigs, finely chopped

Sea salt and freshly ground black pepper

CREAMY POLENTA

4 cups (1 litre) boiling water

1 cup (190 g) fine polenta (white polenta
  if you can find it)

2 tablespoons extra-virgin olive oil

Optional: ½ teaspoon garlic powder
  or 1 garlic clove, crushed

½ cup (60 g) grated kefalograviera
  (see note)

Optional: baby kale leaves and grated
  kefalograviera (see note), to serve

Mixed leaf green salad, to serve

Beetroot, tahini and yoghurt dip, to serve

These turkey meatballs flavoured with fresh coriander are perfect as finger food for parties or, as shown here, a hearty meal served on creamy polenta.

Line a baking tray with baking paper. Using clean hands, mix all the meatball ingredients together in a large bowl.

Lightly oil your hands, then roll the meat mixture into balls the size of large marbles. Place these on the prepared tray, cover, then place in the refrigerator for about 1 hour.

Half an hour before you're ready to serve, make the creamy polenta. Pour the boiling water into a heavy-based saucepan, place over a high heat and season generously with salt. With the water at a rolling boil, whisk in the polenta, then turn the heat down to medium–low and continue whisking until the polenta has thickened.

Cover the pan with a lid, and stir the polenta every 5–10 minutes. Cook for 30 minutes, then remove from the heat. Beat in the olive oil, garlic (if using) and cheese, then cover again to keep warm.

Meanwhile, heat the extra olive oil in a large frying pan over a medium heat and fry the meatballs for about 8 minutes, or until golden on all sides – keep an eye on them. Test one to check it's cooked through – the juices should be clear.

Serve the meatballs with the creamy polenta, a green salad and the Beetroot, tahini and yoghurt dip on page 112, if you like. Scatter over the baby kale and kefalograviera (if using).

NOTE
Kefalograviera is a readily available salty hard pale yellow Greek cheese that melts beautifully. It's used for the classic Greek dish saganaki, and is similar to a gruyere or havarti.

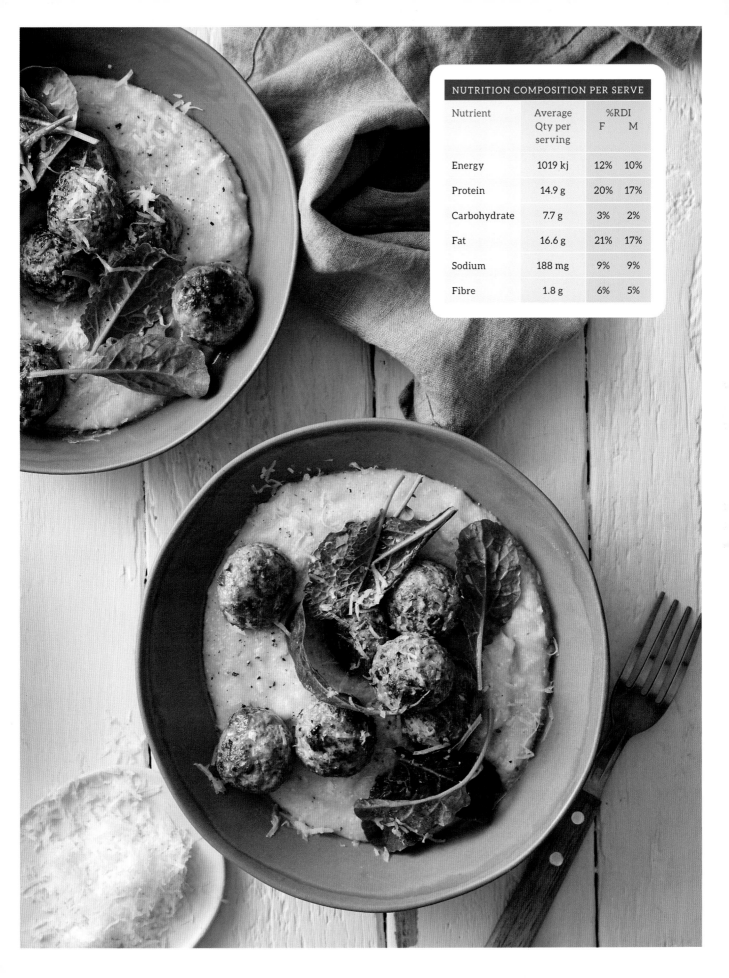

NUTRITION COMPOSITION PER SERVE			
Nutrient	Average Qty per serving	%RDI F	M
Energy	1019 kj	12%	10%
Protein	14.9 g	20%	17%
Carbohydrate	7.7 g	3%	2%
Fat	16.6 g	21%	17%
Sodium	188 mg	9%	9%
Fibre	1.8 g	6%	5%

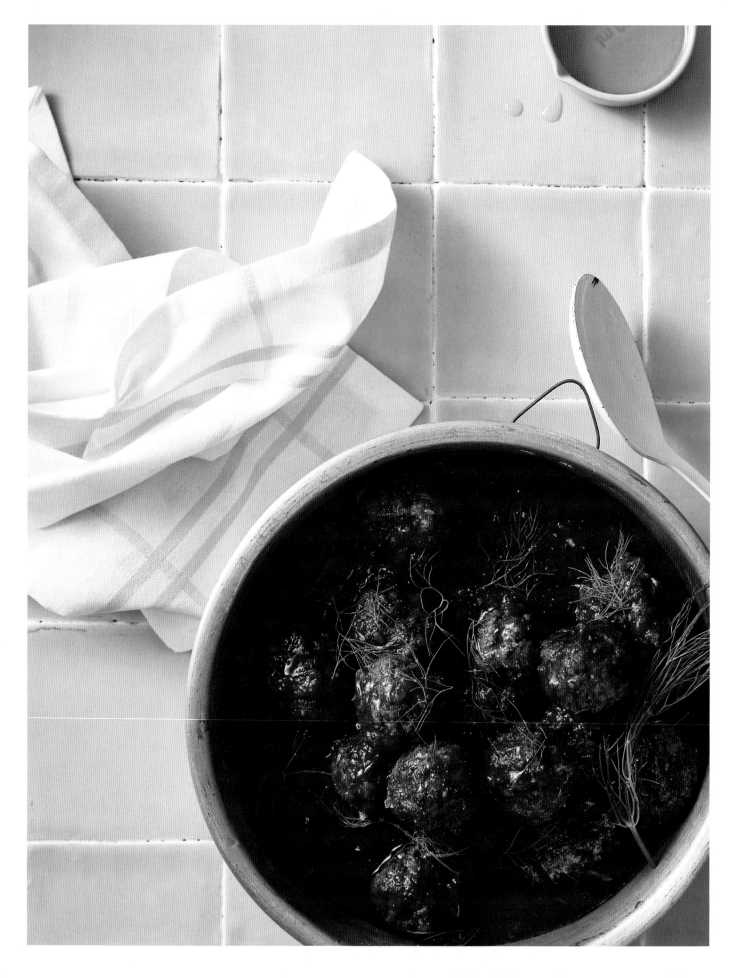

Pork and fennel polpette

2 tablespoons extra-virgin olive oil,
plus extra

MEATBALLS

400 g lean pork mince

1 onion, finely chopped

1 tomato, grated (see tip on page 97)

3 tablespoons gluten-free breadcrumbs

1 teaspoon fennel seeds

¼ fennel bulb, finely chopped

2–3 dill fronds, finely chopped, plus
extra to serve

SAUCE

2 tablespoons extra-virgin olive oil

1 red onion, finely chopped

2 cups (500 ml) purèed tomatoes

4 cups (1 litre) boiling water

Sea salt and freshly ground black pepper

1 fresh bay leaf

½ teaspoon smoked paprika

Fennel seeds have a sweet liquorice-like taste and are rich in anti-inflammatory nutrients. They go well with pork meatballs, and here I have also used some fennel bulb, which gives a softer flavour and moister meatball.

Line a large baking tray with baking paper. Use clean hands to mix all the meatball ingredients together in a bowl with a few good pinches of salt and pepper. Lightly oil your hands to prevent sticking, then roll the mixture into golf ball-sized meatballs. Place on the prepared tray, cover and place in the refrigerator for about 1 hour.

Heat the olive oil in a large non-stick frying pan over a medium–high heat and fry the meatballs for 3–5 minutes, or until lightly golden. Remove and set aside.

To make the sauce, heat the olive oil in a large saucepan over a medium heat and sauté the onion until softened and translucent. Add the tomato and boiling water, then season with salt and pepper. Add the bay leaf and paprika. Simmer for 5 minutes, then carefully add the meatballs and simmer for 20 minutes more.

Garnish the polpette with the extra dill and serve with the Warm broad bean and pea salad (page 137) if you like.

NUTRITION COMPOSITION PER SERVE			
Nutrient	Average Qty per serving	%RDI F	M
Energy	1811 kj	22%	18%
Protein	24 g	33%	27%
Carbohydrate	15.9 g	6%	5%
Fat	30 g	38%	31%
Sodium	493 mg	25%	25%
Fibre	4.9 g	18%	13%

Baked *Mediterranean chicken*

COOKING

1 HOUR

SERVES

6

¼ cup (60 ml) extra-virgin olive oil

1 red onion, chopped

1 × 1.5 kg chicken, cut into 12 pieces
  (ask your butcher to do this for you)

½ cup (125 ml) dry white wine

6 baby red capsicums, halved lengthways
  and deseeded

1½ cups (375 ml) puréed tomato

1 small red chilli, halved, deseeded
  and finely sliced

Optional: 2 tablespoons paprika paste

½ teaspoon smoked paprika

2–3 sage sprigs, leaves picked and
  chopped, plus extra to serve

2 garlic cloves, finely sliced

Sea salt and freshly ground black pepper

4 cups (1 litre) boiling water

100 g pitted kalamata olives

2 x 400 g tins borlotti beans (preferably
  fresh when in season) or butter beans,
  drained and rinsed

TO SERVE

Cos lettuce

Grated dried mizithra cheese, or parmesan

Sourdough bread (see page 106)

This rich and spicy baked chicken combines Mediterranean cultures and is packed with legumes, which extends the meal and adds texture and fibre. Perfect for a family meal on a cold winter's day. You'll see this recipe has the skin on the chicken, but if you'd like to halve the fat content, remove the skin.

Heat the olive oil in a large heavy-based saucepan over a high heat and sauté the onion until softened and translucent. Add the chicken pieces and cook on all sides for about 10 minutes, until lightly golden.

Add the wine to the pan and simmer for about 5 minutes, or until the liquid has evaporated. Add the capsicum and sear on all sides. Add the tomato, chilli, paprika paste (if using), smoked paprika, sage, garlic, salt and pepper and half the boiling water, then reduce the heat to low and simmer for 10 minutes.

Preheat the oven to 180°C and get out a large baking dish.

Add the olives, beans and remaining boiling water to the pan and gently stir. Carefully pour the chicken mixture into the baking dish and bake for 30 minutes. Keep an eye on the liquid levels, and top up with a little extra water if the dish becomes too dry.

When ready to serve, garnish with the extra sage, then take to the table and serve with the cos lettuce, grated cheese for sprinkling and crusty sourdough bread.

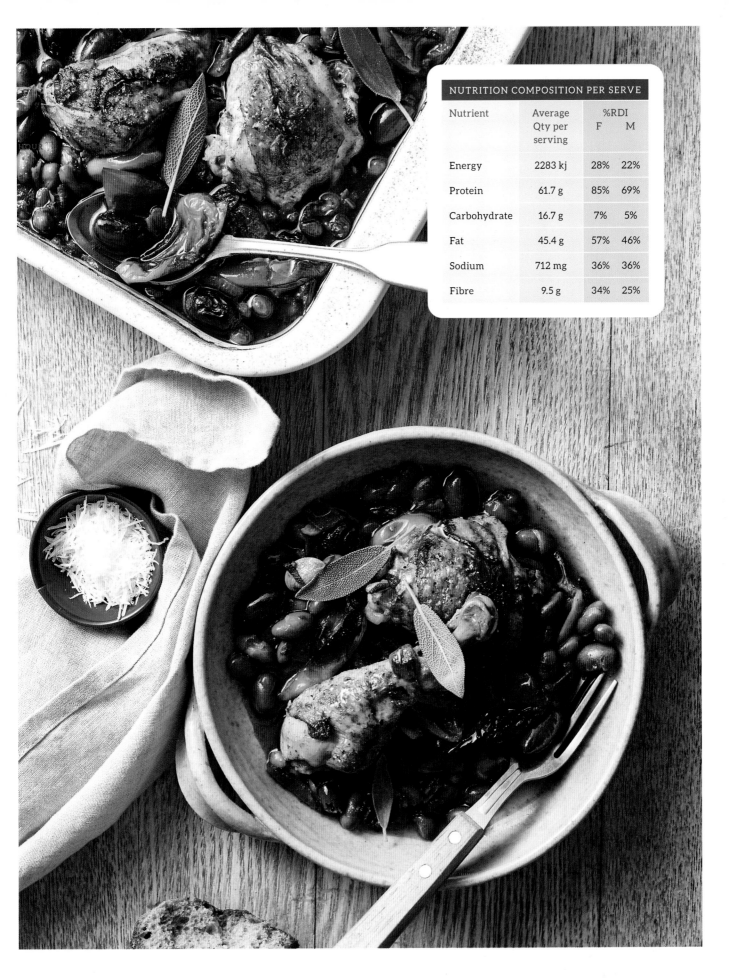

NUTRITION COMPOSITION PER SERVE			
Nutrient	Average Qty per serving	%RDI F	M
Energy	2283 kj	28%	22%
Protein	61.7 g	85%	69%
Carbohydrate	16.7 g	7%	5%
Fat	45.4 g	57%	46%
Sodium	712 mg	36%	36%
Fibre	9.5 g	34%	25%

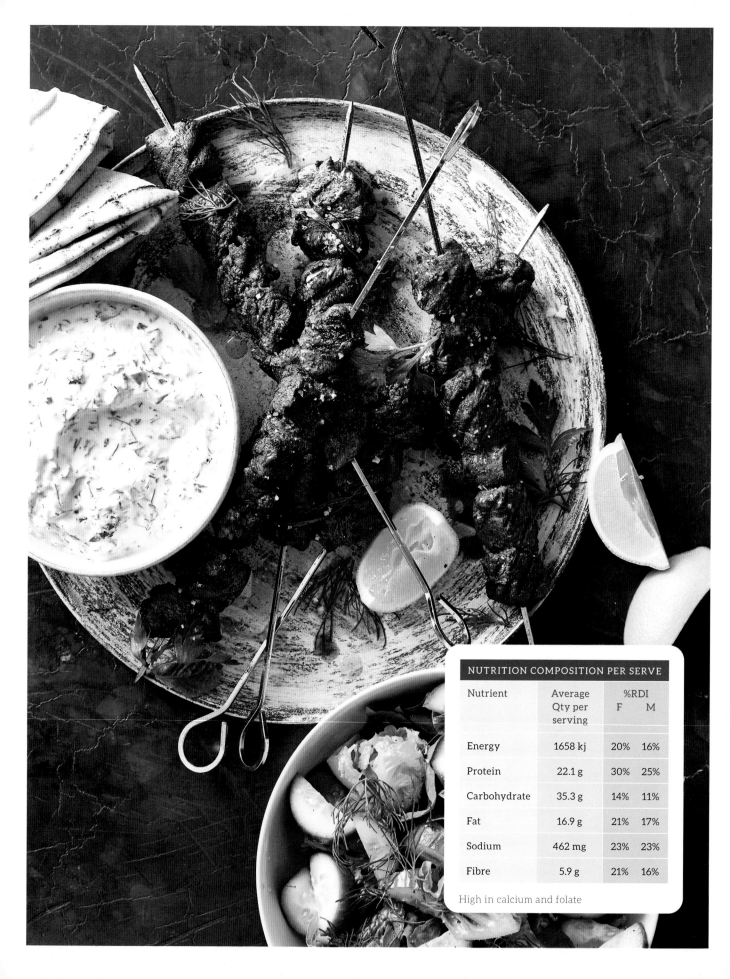

NUTRITION COMPOSITION PER SERVE

Nutrient	Average Qty per serving	%RDI F	M
Energy	1658 kj	20%	16%
Protein	22.1 g	30%	25%
Carbohydrate	35.3 g	14%	11%
Fat	16.9 g	21%	17%
Sodium	462 mg	23%	23%
Fibre	5.9 g	21%	16%

High in calcium and folate

Spicy *lamb souvlaki*

400 g lamb fillets (see intro)

1 tablespoon extra-virgin olive oil,
   for grilling

Fresh herbs and lemon wedges, if on hand

Flatbread of your choosing, to serve
   (I like wholemeal pita bread or the
   Mountain brand of wraps)

Mixed leaf green salad, to serve

SPICE MIX

½ teaspoon cayenne pepper

½ teaspoon cumin powder

1 teaspoon smoked paprika

1 teaspoon dried oregano

Sea salt and freshly ground black pepper

HERB YOGHURT

1 cup (250 g) thick Greek-style yoghurt

1 tablespoon extra-virgin olive oil

1 tablespoon finely chopped
   flat-leaf parsley

1 tablespoon finely chopped mint

1 tablespoon finely chopped dill

¼ preserved lemon rind, finely diced

This classic Greek lamb souvlaki is basted in aromatic spices like cumin to add an Eastern Mediterranean twist and anti-inflammatory nutrients. These fillets can be prepared whole or cut into 4–5 pieces, then threaded onto a skewer for cooking (souvlaki style).

Combine all the spices for the spice mixture together in a small bowl and add a good pinch of salt and pepper. Rub the lamb fillets with the olive oil, then sprinkle over the spice mix and toss to coat evenly.

Mix together all the herb yoghurt ingredients in a bowl and set aside.

Grill the spiced lamb on a lightly oiled hot plate or chargrill pan over a medium heat, or cook on the barbecue for a few minutes on each side until cooked to your liking.

Garnish the souvlaki with the fresh herbs and lemon wedges, if on hand, then serve on any style of flatbread you like with a spoonful of herb yoghurt and a green salad or the gluten-free tabbouleh on page 151.

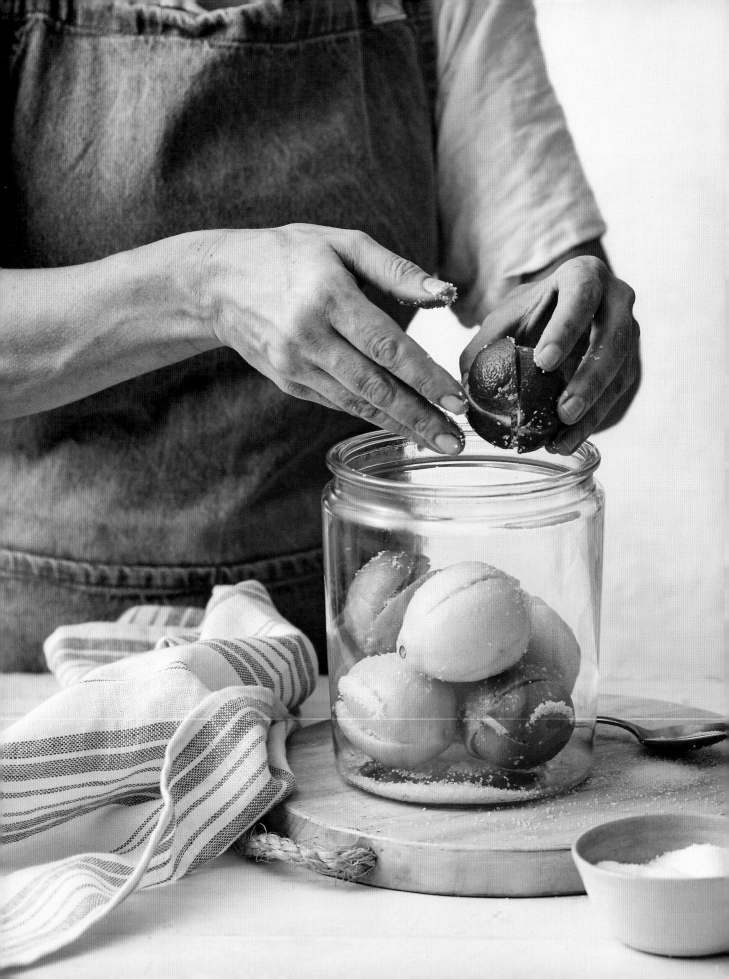

Preserved *lemons and limes*

COOKING
30 MINUTES

YIELDS A
1 LITRE JAR

4–6 lemons and/or limes

½ cup (150 g) cooking salt

1 litre-capacity pickling jar with lid

4–6 fresh bay leaves

1 teaspoon fennel seeds

2 cups (500 ml) freshly squeezed lemon
   or lime juice (depending on which fruit
   you're preserving)

Adding preserved lemons and limes to a dish gives it an intense citrus flavour. Preserving tempers the bitterness of the citrus. It's sometimes hard to find in shops so why not make your own, especially when you have extra lemons or limes on hand. I use preserved lemons and limes in the Cauliflower steaks with turmeric yoghurt on page 104, Beetroot, tahini and yoghurt dip on page 112, Grilled calamari on cavolo nero pesto on page 168 and Herb yoghurt on page 205.

Step 1: Wash the fruit and cut lengthways almost into quarters; only cut part way through, leaving the base intact. Place in a freezer bag and freeze overnight. The next day, thaw the fruit (this softens the peel). Alternatively, you can boil the whole fruit in a large saucepan for 30 minutes until the skins soften a little, then cool and quarter them part way.

Step 2: Pack the centre of each fruit with plenty of salt, then place in the jar. Add the bay leaves and fennel seeds between the lemons and/or limes.

Step 3: Fill the jar right to the top with the lemon or lime juice, or half of each for mixed citrus, then seal and store in a cool dark place for 4–6 weeks.

Step 4: When ready to use, remove and discard the flesh and pith and use the softened rind in recipes.

NUTRITION COMPOSITION PER SERVE

Nutrient	Average Qty per serving	%RDI F	M
Energy	112 kj	1%	1%
Protein	0.58 g	1%	1%
Carbohydrate	1.75 g	1%	1%
Fat	0.19 g	<1%	<1%
Sodium	668 mg	33%	33%
Fibre	2.43 g	9%	6%

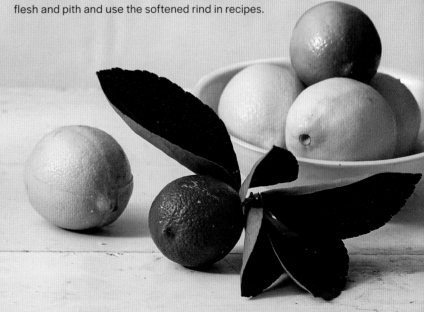

Kleftiko lamb fillets

COOKING
50 MINUTES

SERVES
4–6

2 bullhorn or long red mild chillies

Extra-virgin olive oil

500 g lamb fillets

¼ teaspoon ground cumin

2 garlic cloves, crushed

Sea salt and freshly ground black pepper

2–3 rosemary sprigs, leaves picked and chopped

1 red onion, cut into wedges

1–2 bunches broccolini, trimmed

Optional: 4 thin slices of kefalograviera (see note on page 198) or feta

2–3 dill sprigs, chopped, and lemon wedges, if on hand

Greek salad, to serve

GARLIC YOGHURT

200 g thick Greek-style yoghurt

1 garlic clove, crushed

1 tablespoon extra-virgin olive oil

Ground cumin

The Greek word kleftiko means stolen, and the story behind this method of cooking lamb is that shepherds would occasionally steal someone else's lamb and cook it on coals in a hole in the ground covered with rocks so the owner wouldn't recognise their animal. Today we cook the lamb by wrapping the meat in foil. It is a versatile way of cooking that keeps the meat deliciously moist.

Preheat the oven to 200°C. Line a baking tray with baking paper. Place the chillies on the prepared tray and roast for 20 minutes, or until really soft. Allow to cool, then deseed and slice.

Rub some olive oil all over the lamb, then add the cumin, garlic, salt, pepper and half the chopped rosemary and rub all over the lamb before covering and refrigerating for 30 minutes.

Preheat the oven to 180°C. Heat a large chargrill pan and drizzle with olive oil. Sear the lamb on each side, then set aside. Lightly chargrill the onion until softened, then set aside. Chargrill the broccolini for 2–3 minutes on each side, then remove from the heat.

Place four 15 cm squares of foil on a large baking tray so the base of the tray is completely covered and the foil hangs over the sides of the tray (use more foil if needed) – enough to make a parcel with. Spread the grilled broccolini around the foil, top with the onion, then add a layer of the chilli and crumble over the cheese. Place the lamb fillets on top, season with salt and pepper and garnish with the remaining rosemary. Seal the foil parcel by folding up the sides and pinching them together. Bake for 20 minutes.

Make the garlic yoghurt by mixing the yoghurt, garlic and olive oil in a bowl. Season with salt and a sprinkle of ground cumin to taste.

Serve the lamb kleftiko in the foil with the dill and lemon wedges, if on hand, and a Greek salad and the garlic yoghurt.

Nutrient	Average Qty per serving	%RDI F	M
Energy	1621 kj	20%	16%
Protein	34.5 g	47%	38%
Carbohydrate	15 g	6%	5%
Fat	19.9 g	25%	20%
Sodium	267 mg	13%	13%
Fibre	4.9 g	18%	13%

NUTRITION COMPOSITION PER SERVE

High in iron, selenium and vitamin C

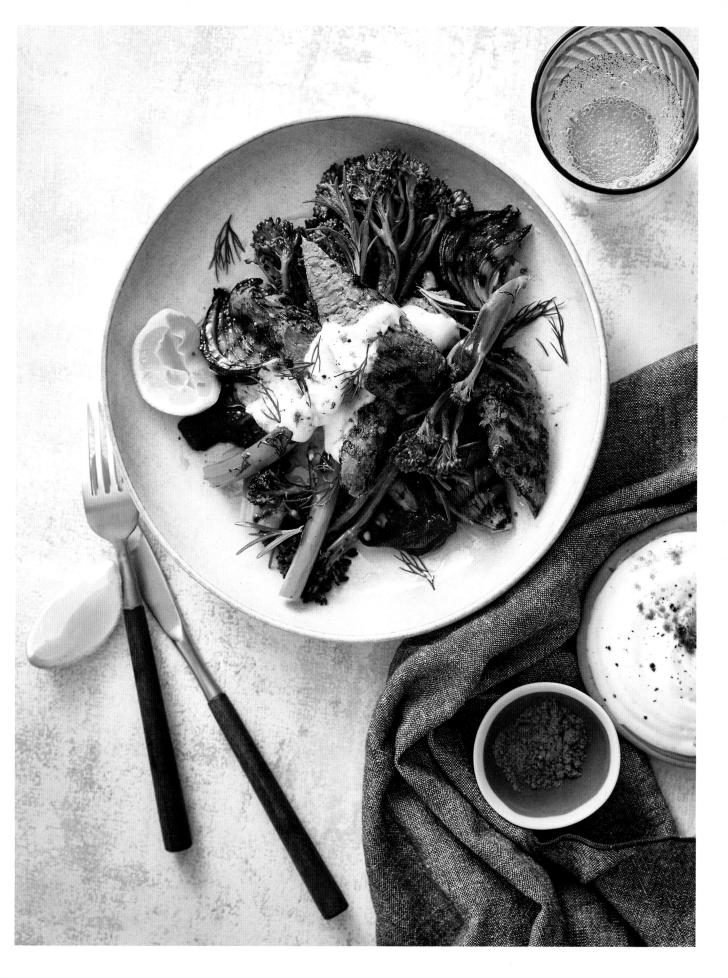

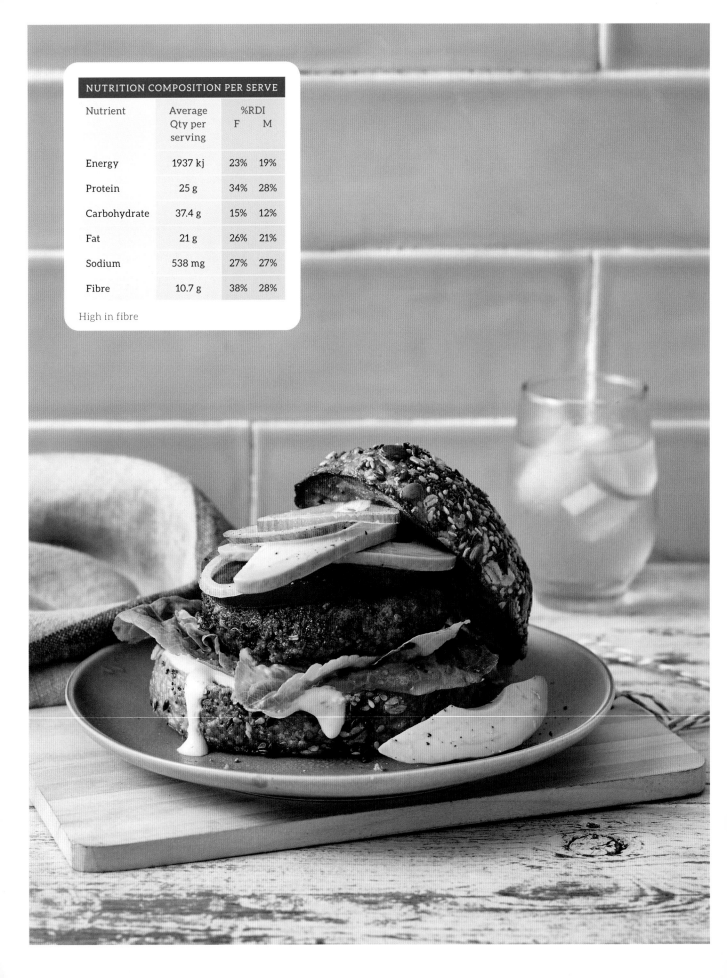

Nutrient	Average Qty per serving	%RDI	
		F	M
Energy	1937 kj	23%	19%
Protein	25 g	34%	28%
Carbohydrate	37.4 g	15%	12%
Fat	21 g	26%	21%
Sodium	538 mg	27%	27%
Fibre	10.7 g	38%	28%

NUTRITION COMPOSITION PER SERVE

High in fibre

Meat and mushroom **burger**

300 g pork and veal mince

200 g mushrooms, cleaned and minced
  (use a food processor for this)

1 red onion, grated

1 tomato, grated (see tip on page 97)

1 tablespoon finely chopped flat-leaf
  parsley

½ teaspoon dried oregano

½ teaspoon dried rosemary

2 tablespoons extra-virgin olive oil,
  plus extra for grilling

Sea salt and freshly ground black pepper

1 egg, lightly beaten

3 tablespoons gluten-free
  (or regular) breadcrumbs

Optional: ½ teaspoon chilli flakes

TO SERVE

6–8 gluten-free or wholegrain burger buns

Optional: thick Greek-style yoghurt

1 avocado, sliced

1 baby cos lettuce, leaves separated

1 large tomato, thickly sliced

1 small red onion, finely sliced

This burger is made with a 60:40 ratio of meat (pork and veal mince) to mushrooms, making it a great option for meat eaters who are keen to up their veggie intake. If you aren't keen on serving your burgers in a bun, you can serve it with the Fresh tomato salad on page 141, some crispy cos lettuce and a dollop of the Herb yoghurt on page 205. It's also great served with some beetroot, butter bean and yoghurt sauce (see tip below).

Line a baking tray with baking paper. Place the meat in a large bowl with the minced mushroom, onion, tomato, parsley, oregano and rosemary. Add the olive oil and salt and pepper, then mix everything together well with clean hands. Add the egg and breadcrumbs and mix well before rolling into golf ball-sized portions. Flatten these into six patties (or eight slightly smaller ones) and place on the prepared tray. Cover and refrigerate for 30 minutes to 1 hour.

When ready to cook, heat a chargrill pan on the stovetop and drizzle with the extra olive oil. Add the patties and cook until browned on both sides. To check that the burgers are cooked through, press gently on one with a spatula – if the juices run clear, it's ready. Alternatively, you can cut one open and check.

Serve each burger in a bun spread with yoghurt (if using). Top with a drizzle of yoghurt and some avocado, cos lettuce, tomato and onion.

TIP

To make a beetroot, butter bean and yoghurt sauce, add 1 large or 2 small roasted or boiled beetroots to a food processor with 1 x 400 g tin of butter beans (drained and rinsed), 1 garlic clove, 1 tablespoon of extra-virgin olive oil and 2 tablespoons of Greek-style yoghurt. Blend until creamy, then season with salt and pepper. You can also use this instead of avocado on the burger bun.

Marinated *pork cutlets* with roasted apples

COOKING
20
MINUTES

SERVES
2

2 x 250 g bone-in pork cutlets, fat trimmed

2 tablespoons extra-virgin olive oil, plus extra for cooking

Sea salt and freshly ground black pepper

1 teaspoon dried thyme

1–2 teaspoons ground coriander

1 teaspoon finely chopped sage

½ fennel bulb, sliced, plus fronds

Green salad, to serve

ROASTED APPLES

2 royal gala apples, cored and quartered

1 tablespoon raw sugar

Ground nutmeg, to serve

These grilled pork cutlets with chargrilled fennel make a perfect autumn day lunch accompanied by a glass of chianti wine.

Rub the pork cutlets with the olive oil and season with salt and pepper, thyme, coriander and sage. Rub these seasonings all over the pork, then cover and refrigerate for a few hours until ready to cook.

When ready to cook, preheat the oven to 180°C. Line a baking tray with baking paper. Arrange the apple quarters on the prepared tray, then sprinkle with the sugar and bake for 20 minutes, or until softened.

Meanwhile, drizzle some olive oil on a grill plate over a medium–high heat. Add the pork chops and cook for 5 minutes or more on each side (according to your preference).

Season the sliced fennel with salt and pepper, then add it to the oiled grill plate and char slightly on each side until it softens a little.

Sprinkle a few pinches of nutmeg over the roasted apples. Divide the pork chops, grilled fennel and apples between two plates, garnish with the fennel fronds, then serve with a green salad.

NUTRITION COMPOSITION PER SERVE			
Nutrient	Average Qty per serving	%RDI F	M
Energy	2223 kj	27%	22%
Protein	49.6 g	68%	55%
Carbohydrate	30 g	12%	9%
Fat	22.5 g	28%	23%
Sodium	261 mg	13%	13%
Fibre	5.7 g	20%	15%

High in thiamine (vitamin B1)
and niacin (vitamin B3)

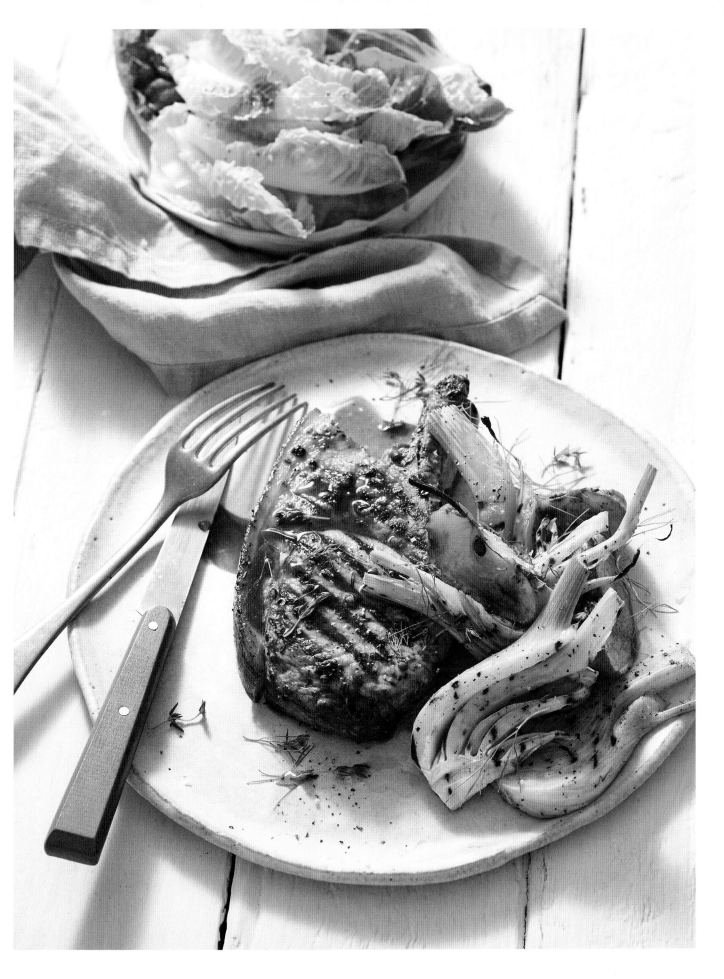

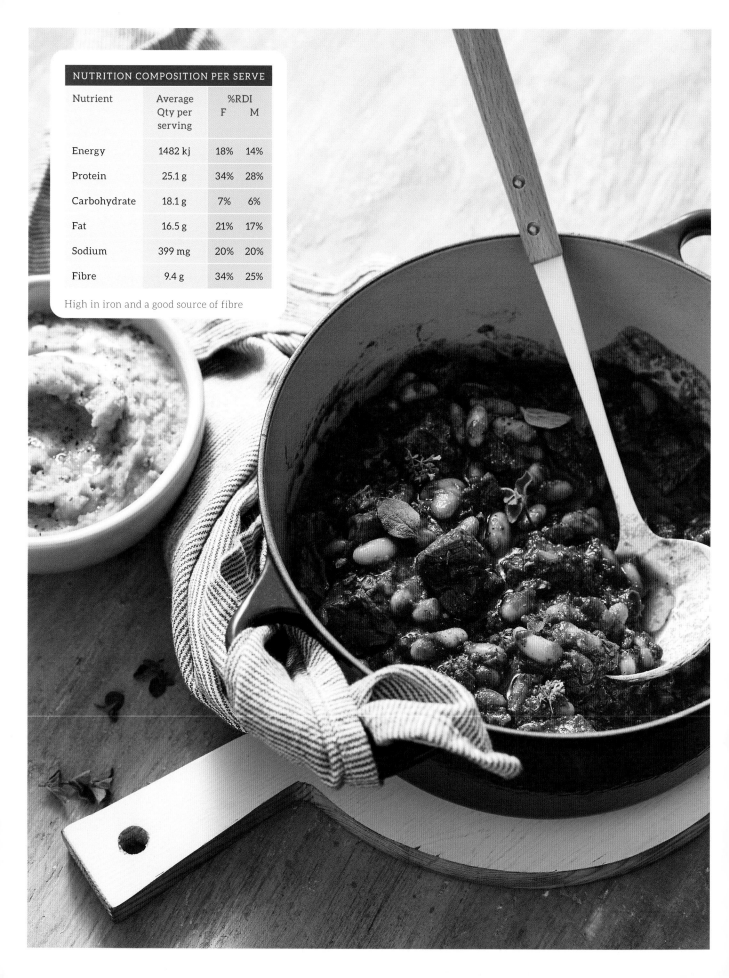

NUTRITION COMPOSITION PER SERVE

Nutrient	Average Qty per serving	%RDI F	M
Energy	1482 kj	18%	14%
Protein	25.1 g	34%	28%
Carbohydrate	18.1 g	7%	6%
Fat	16.5 g	21%	17%
Sodium	399 mg	20%	20%
Fibre	9.4 g	34%	25%

High in iron and a good source of fibre

Beef cassoulet

COOKING

2 HOURS + 30 MINUTES

SERVES

6

⅓ cup (80 ml) extra-virgin olive oil

1 onion, finely chopped

500 g beef rump, cut into 2 cm pieces

½ cup (125 ml) red wine

1 small red chilli, halved, deseeded
  and finely chopped

2 garlic cloves, finely chopped

1 red capsicum, deseeded and diced

½ fennel bulb, diced

1 celery stalk, diced

½ teaspoon dried thyme

½ teaspoon fennel seeds or celery seeds

½ teaspoon ground coriander

½ teaspoon dried or fresh oregano leaves

1 x 400 g tin crushed tomatoes

1 cup (250 ml) puréed tomato

4 cups (1 litre) boiling water, plus extra,
  if needed

2 x 400 g tins cannellini beans, drained

Leafy salad, to serve

SWEET POTATO MASH

1 kg white sweet potato, cut into
  2 cm pieces

2 garlic cloves, unpeeled

2 tablespoons extra-virgin olive oil

½ teaspoon dried or fresh thyme leaves

Sea salt and freshly ground black pepper

This hearty dish of slow-cooked beef with cannellini beans and creamy sweet potato mash is the perfect comfort food on a cold winter's day. The cut of meat determines the cooking time, fillets cook faster than rump or shoulder cuts.

Heat some olive oil in a large flameproof casserole dish over a medium heat and sauté the onion until softened and translucent. Add the beef and sear on all sides. Pour in the wine and simmer until the alcohol has mostly evaporated, then add the chilli, garlic, capsicum, fennel, celery and herbs. Sauté for 5–10 minutes, then add the tinned and puréed tomatoes and 2 cups (500 ml) of boiling water.

Simmer the cassoulet on a low heat for 2 hours, then remove a piece of meat from the dish and check it. If it's still tough, add a little more boiling water and continue to simmer for another 20 minutes.

Meanwhile, preheat the oven to 180°C and spread the sweet potato and garlic cloves on a baking tray lined with baking paper. Roast for 20 minutes until soft, then transfer the sweet potato to a large bowl. Squeeze the roasted garlic into the bowl, discarding the skins. Roughly mash, then drizzle with the olive oil and season well with the thyme, salt and pepper. Cover to keep warm.

Add the cannellini beans to the casserole and another 2 cups (500 ml) of boiling water, and simmer for another 15 minutes, checking that the dish has enough water.

Serve the cassoulet with the sweet potato mash or Creamy polenta (see page 198) and a leafy salad.

Chicken on a spit

1 x 375 ml drink can, half-filled with any of the following: lemon iced tea, beer, lemon-flavoured mineral water, soda water with lemon juice

1 x 1.5 kg chicken

½ cup (125 ml) extra-virgin olive oil, plus extra

1 teaspoon oregano leaves

1 teaspoon dried or finely chopped rosemary leaves

½ teaspoon sweet paprika

½ teaspoon chilli flakes

Sea salt and freshly ground black pepper

Juice 2 lemons (reserve a lemon half)

1 bunch (250 g) rainbow Dutch carrots, peeled

500 g royal blue baby potatoes, halved (preferably unpeeled)

2 red onions, quartered

4 or 5 garlic cloves, unpeeled

1 cup (250 ml) boiling water

This way of cooking a whole chicken has become popular as it is easy and produces moist, tasty results. My husband, Savvas, put this recipe together and it reminds us of a chicken souvla (chicken on a spit), only this one stands on a can in the oven!

Preheat the oven to 190°C. Stand a can – half-filled with the liquid of your choice – in the middle of a large roasting tin. Check the oven to make sure the shelves will accommodate a chicken standing upright.

Wash the chicken under running water, then pat dry with kitchen paper. Rub with the olive oil and half of the oregano, rosemary, paprika, chilli flakes, salt and pepper.

Place the reserved juiced lemon half inside the chicken cavity, then carefully stand the chicken on the upright can in the tin.

Arrange the vegetables and garlic cloves around the chicken, then season well with the remaining herbs and spices. Drizzle over some extra olive oil, then pour the boiling water into the tin and carefully place it in the oven.

Roast for 30–45 minutes, or until the chicken is cooked through and the juices run clear when the thickest part of a thigh is pierced with a knife.

Serve the chicken with the roasted vegetables and the Sautéed wild greens (see page 89).

NUTRITION COMPOSITION PER SERVE			
Nutrient	Average Qty per serving	%RDI F	M
Energy	3021 kj	37%	29%
Protein	47.5 g	65%	53%
Carbohydrate	14.5 g	6%	5%
Fat	51.7 g	65%	53%
Sodium	233 mg	12%	12%
Fibre	5.3 g	19%	14%

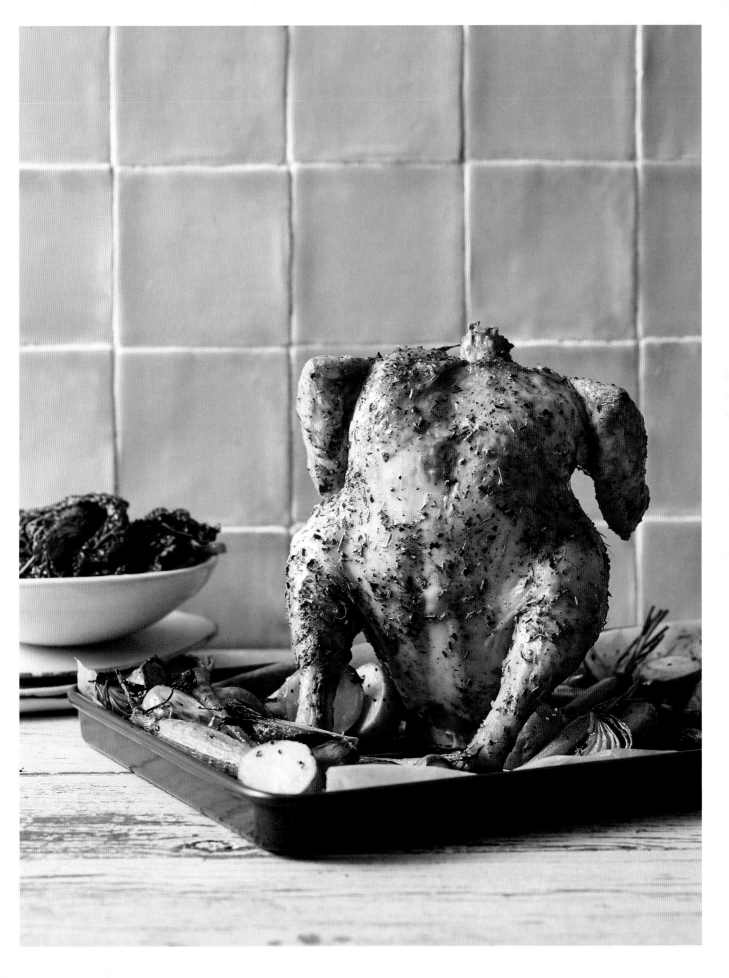

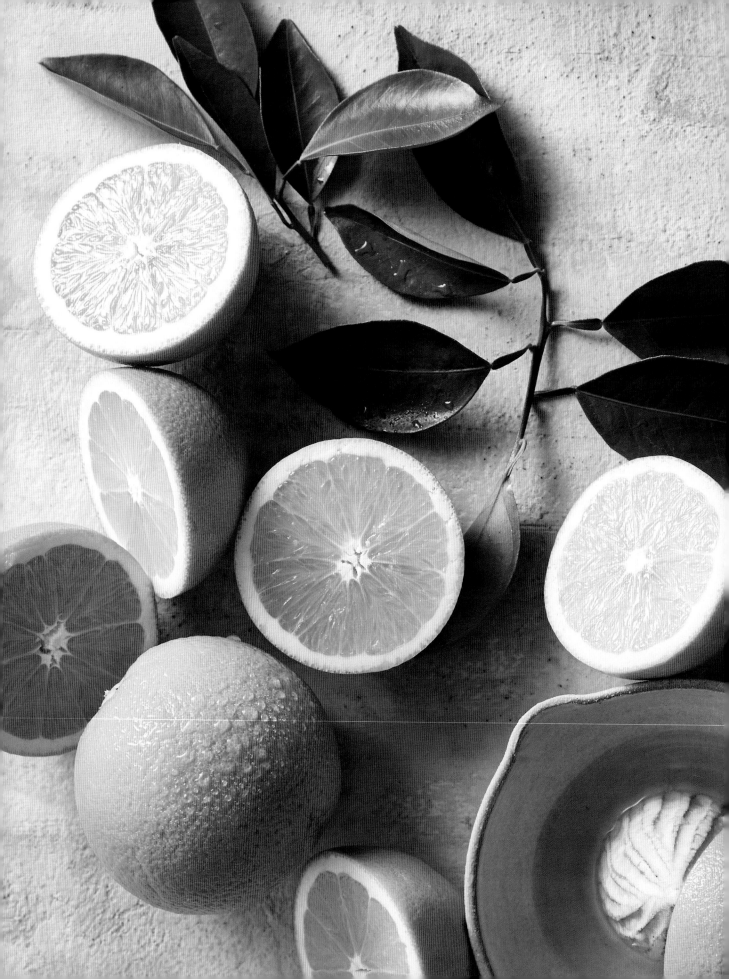

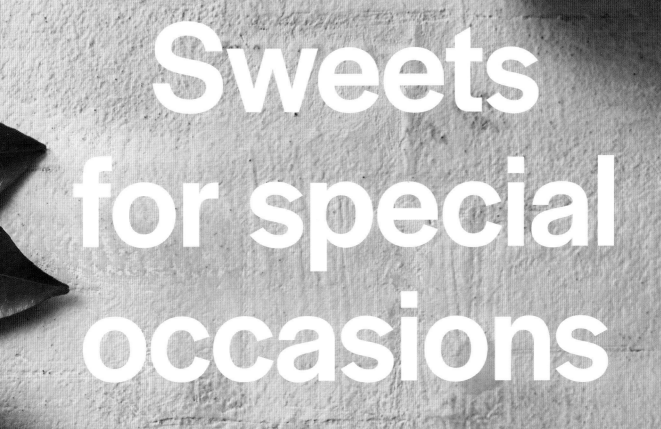

Sweets
for special
occasions

———

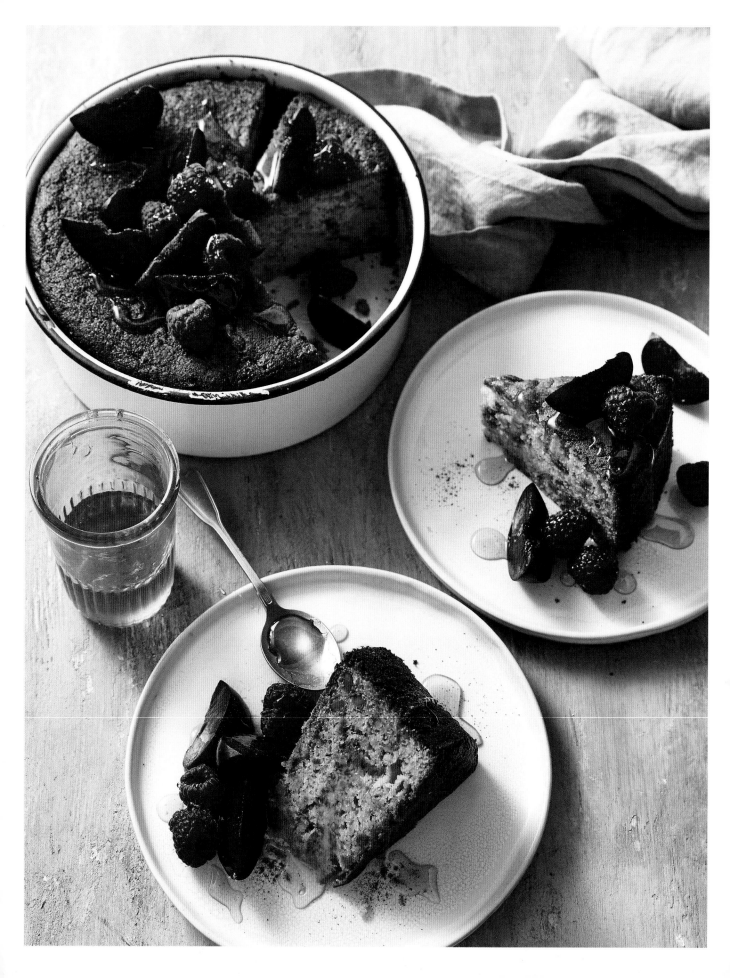

Flourless *orange and date* cake

COOKING
50
MINUTES

SERVES
8

1½ cups (180 g) gluten-free plain flour

2 teaspoons baking powder

½ cup (50 g) almond meal

½ cup (125 g) honey, plus extra to serve

3 eggs, separated

3 tablespoons thick Greek-style yoghurt,
plus extra to serve

1 teaspoon finely chopped sage

Zest and juice 1 orange (or blood orange,
if available)

Fine sea salt

100 ml extra-virgin olive oil (use a light
variety for baking), plus extra for greasing

8 pitted dates (100 g), soaked in boiling
water, then drained and finely chopped

½ cup (50 g) crushed walnuts

½ teaspoon ground cinnamon, plus extra
for dusting

Optional: raspberries, strawberries
and plum wedges, to serve

A treat you can enjoy with little guilt. Yoghurt, citrus, dried fruit and nuts are all featured in this moist cake.

Preheat the oven to 170°C and lightly grease a 20 cm round cake tin with olive oil. Line the base and side of the tin with baking paper and set aside.

Sift the flour and baking powder into a mixing bowl, then add the almond meal. Set aside.

In another large mixing bowl, combine the honey and egg yolks and beat with an electric mixer until the mixture is thick and pale. Beat in the yoghurt, sage and zest and juice from the orange. Add a pinch of salt and gradually drizzle in the olive oil as you continue to beat.

Beat the sifted flours into the mixture on a low speed. Once combined, add the chopped dates, walnuts and cinnamon.

Beat the egg whites in a clean bowl until soft peaks form, then gently fold into the batter. Pour the batter into the prepared tin, then bake for 50 minutes.

Insert a skewer into the centre of the cake – if it comes out clean, the cake is cooked; if batter remains on the skewer, cook for a few minutes more.

Cool the cake in the tin for 10 minutes, then turn out and transfer to a wire rack to cool completely.

Dust the cake with the extra cinnamon, then serve with the yoghurt, berries, plums and honey (if using).

NUTRITION COMPOSITION PER SERVE			
Nutrient	Average Qty per serving	%RDI F	M
Energy	1546 kj	19%	15%
Protein	6.3 g	9%	7%
Carbohydrate	36.7 g	15%	11%
Fat	21.8 g	27%	22%
Sodium	79 mg	4%	4%
Fibre	2.4 g	9%	6%

Healthy Heart **pasteli**

These healthy bars are a perfect snack with your morning coffee or for that afternoon pick-me-up. Varying the amount of honey changes the consistency – more honey means chewier bars.

1 cup (250 g) honey

2 cups (300 g) sesame seeds

⅔ cups (100 g) pumpkin seeds

3 tablespoons (30 g) flaxseeds

2 tablespoons dried cranberries

2 tablespoons dried blueberries
  or currants

1 teaspoon ground cinnamon

½ teaspoon allspice

NUTRITION COMPOSITION PER SERVE

Nutrient	Average Qty per serving	%RDI	
		F	M
Energy	1016 kj	12%	10%
Protein	6.4 g	9%	7%
Carbohydrate	21.9 g	9%	7%
Fat	14.3 g	18%	15%
Sodium	10 mg	1%	1%
Fibre	3 g	11%	8%

Line a 20 x 30 cm lamington tin with baking paper. Heat the honey in a saucepan over a medium heat until it just starts to bubble, then simmer for 5 minutes. Remove from the heat.

Combine the seeds and toast in a dry heavy-based saucepan over a low heat for 5–10 minutes, or until the sesame seeds start to brown. Add the dried berries, cinnamon and allspice and continue to toast for a few minutes.

Pour the hot honey into the seed mixture and stir for 5–6 minutes, or until the mixture starts to stick to the spoon. Pour into the prepared tin, place another layer of baking paper over the top, then roll flat with a rolling pin. Remove the top layer of paper. Allow to cool and set for 30 minutes.

Cut into small squares or diamond shapes, then store in an airtight container for up to 2 weeks with sheets of baking paper between layers to prevent them sticking together.

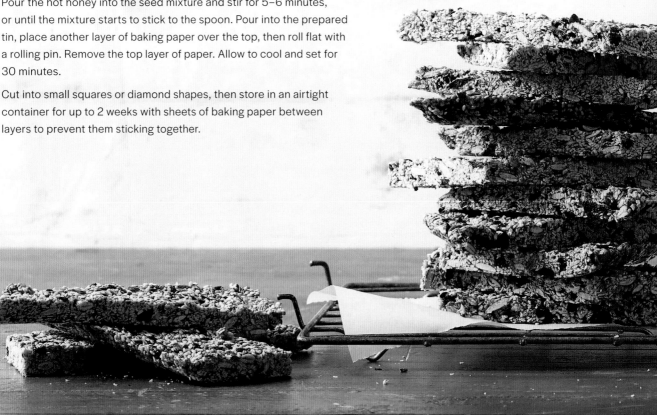

Hazelnut biscuits

COOKING **18** MINUTES

MAKES **40**

These chewy hazelnut biscuits are perfect with an espresso.

3 egg whites

1½ cups (330 g) raw sugar

3 cups (270 g) hazelnut meal

1 teaspoon ground cinnamon

1 teaspoon vanilla sugar

1 tablespoon mastiha or Cointreau liqueur (see note)

200 g hazelnuts, roughly crushed

NUTRITION COMPOSITION PER SERVE			
Nutrient	Average Qty per serving	%RDI	
		F	M
Energy	761 kj	9%	7%
Protein	3.3 g	5%	4%
Carbohydrate	16.2 g	6%	5%
Fat	11.4 g	14%	12%
Sodium	10 mg	1%	1%
Fibre	2 g	7%	5%

Preheat the oven to 180°C. Line a baking tray (you may need two depending on how large your trays are) with baking paper.

Beat the egg whites using electric beaters in a mixing bowl until soft peaks form. Add the sugar and continue beating until the sugar is well incorporated into the egg white.

In another large bowl, combine the hazelnut meal, cinnamon, vanilla sugar and liqueur. Fold the egg white mixture into the hazelnut mixture.

Drop tablespoonfuls of the mixture into the crushed hazelnuts and gently roll to coat. The balls should be walnut-sized pieces. (If you prefer, you can mix the crushed hazelnuts into the dough for all-through crunch).

Place the biscuits on the prepared tray(s), leaving a little space around each biscuit – they do spread a little during cooking. Bake for 16–18 minutes, or until the biscuits are golden. Transfer the trays to a wire rack and allow to cool. These biscuits will be very soft when they come out of the oven, but will harden as they cool. Store in an airtight container for up to 1 week.

NOTE

Mastiha is a thick and syrupy liqueur. A vanilla liqueur or sugar syrup is a good substitute.

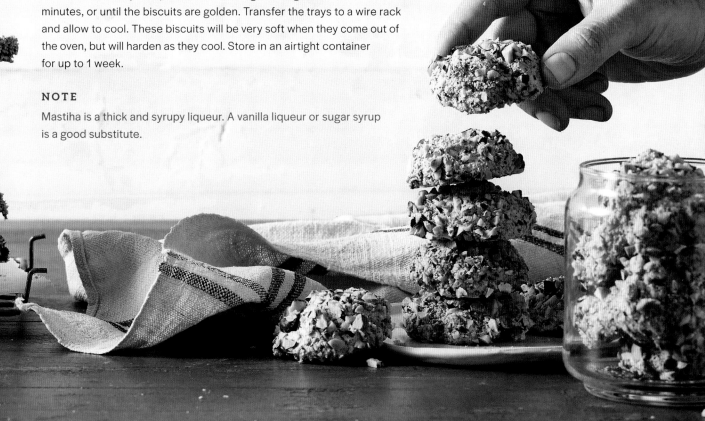

Lemony yoghurt tart

Extra-virgin olive oil, for greasing

Fresh berries, to serve

BASE

½ cup (75 g) almonds

¼ cup (35 g) pistachios

¼ cup (35 g) hazelnuts

1 teaspoon ground cinnamon

Fine sea salt

3 pitted dates, soaked in boiling water
    for 10 minutes

3 dried figs (see note), soaked in boiling
    water for 10 minutes

FILLING

3 eggs

½ cup (115 g) caster sugar

80 g honey

Zest and juice 2 lemons

½ teaspoon ground nutmeg, plus extra
    for dusting

1 cup (250 g) thick Greek-style yoghurt

An impressive-looking tart for that special occasion. Best of all, it's delicious and guilt-free, as the base is full of healthy nuts and the filling is made from Greek-style yoghurt and honey.

Preheat the oven to 180°C. Lightly grease a 20 cm fluted tart tin with a removable base with olive oil. Line the base with baking paper.

Place the nuts, cinnamon and a pinch of salt in a food processor and pulse until you have a coarse mixture (the base should have texture and crunch). Drain the soaked dates and figs, add and blend again until the mixture starts to stick together.

Press the base mixture into the base and side of the tart tin – ensuring it is evenly spread. Bake for 10–12 minutes, or until the base starts to brown around the edge, then set aside.

To make the filling, lower the oven temperature to 150°C. Whisk the eggs and sugar until well combined, add the honey and lemon zest and gradually add the lemon juice while whisking. Add the nutmeg and yoghurt and whisk. Pour this mixture on top of the nut base and spread out evenly. Bake in the centre of the oven for 30 minutes, or until the filling is set and the middle is still a little wobbly. Allow to cool in the tin.

Eat on the day of cooking if you like a custard consistency. Alternatively, place in the fridge for a couple of hours or overnight for a firmer consistency. Decorate with the berries and a dusting of extra nutmeg before serving.

NOTE

You can also use 7 dried dates rather than a mixture of dates and figs if you don't have dried figs.

NUTRITION COMPOSITION PER SERVE			
Nutrient	Average Qty per serving	%RDI	
		F	M
Energy	921 kj	11%	9%
Protein	10.3 g	14%	11%
Carbohydrate	8.3 g	3%	3%
Fat	16 g	20%	16%
Sodium	127 mg	6%	6%
Fibre	2.6 g	9%	7%

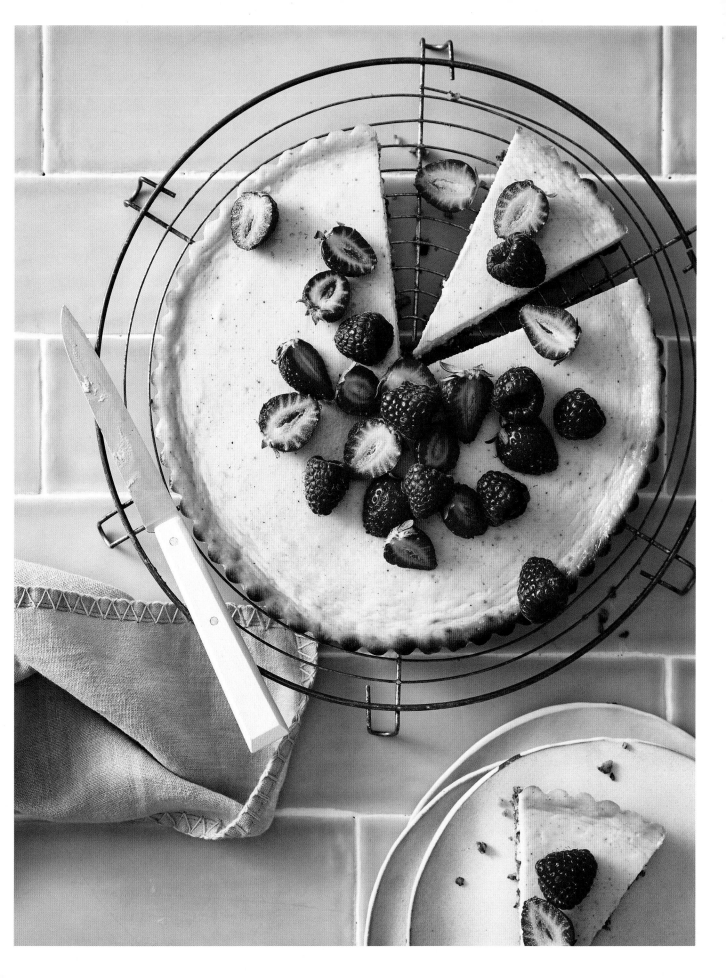

Pistachio baklava

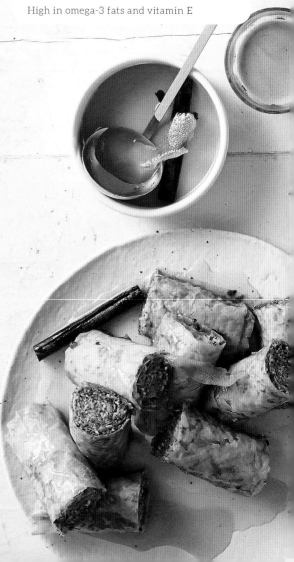

COOKING
40 MINUTES

MAKES
20

A classic dessert of crushed nuts, thin filo pastry and honey, in this variation I've swapped out half the walnuts for pistachios and spiced it up with cinnamon, nutmeg and cloves.

1 cup (140 g) pistachios, finely chopped

1 cup (100 g) walnuts, finely chopped

¾ cup (100 g) sesame seeds

½ teaspoon ground cinnamon, plus extra for dusting

¼ teaspoon ground cloves

¼ teaspoon ground nutmeg

2 tablespoons raw sugar

180 g (½ pack or 10 sheets) frozen filo pastry, thawed

¼ cup (60 ml) extra-virgin olive oil, for brushing, plus extra for greasing

SYRUP

1½ cups (375 ml) water

1 cup (220 g) raw sugar

Zest 1 lemon

1 tablespoon lemon juice

1 cinnamon stick

3–4 cloves

2 tablespoons honey

Nutrient	Average Qty per serving	%RDI	
		F	M
Energy	872 kj	11%	9%
Protein	4.1 g	6%	5%
Carbohydrate	19 g	8%	6%
Fat	12.9 g	16%	13%
Sodium	55 mg	3%	3%
Fibre	1.8 g	6%	5%

NUTRITION COMPOSITION PER SERVE

High in omega-3 fats and vitamin E

Preheat the oven to 180°C. Grease a 20 x 30 cm lamington tin with olive oil. Combine the pistachios, walnuts, sesame seeds, spices and sugar in a bowl.

Spread the thawed filo sheets out on a damp tea towel (this will prevent them from drying out while you work with them). Brush one pastry sheet lightly with the oil, then place another sheet on top and brush that lightly with oil. Sprinkle one-fifth of the nut and seed mixture over the oiled filo, then tightly roll up the pastry from the short side until you have a long cigar shape. Repeat these steps until you have five baklava pastry rolls. Place each roll in the prepared tin, then brush them with olive oil to prevent them from drying out in the oven. Cut each roll into four equal pieces.

Bake for 30 minutes until golden – sprinkling a little water over the pastry now and then to stop it from curling and cracking during baking.

Meanwhile, make the syrup by bringing the water, sugar, lemon zest and juice, cinnamon stick and cloves to the boil in a small saucepan. Reduce the heat and simmer for 5 minutes. Add the honey and simmer for a further 5 minutes, or until the syrup starts to thicken a little.

Once the baklava is cooked, leave it in the tin and pour the syrup all over the hot baklava. Allow to stand for 15 minutes so the syrup soaks in.

Serve the baklava hot or cold, dusted with extra cinnamon. Store in an airtight container for up to 1 week.

Baklava clusters

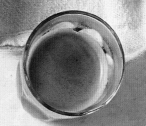

COOKING **45** MINUTES

SERVES **15**

This is a variation on the pistachio baklava opposite. It uses most of the same ingredients, but here they are made into delicious little clusters that can be eaten with yoghurt and fresh berries for a filling breakfast, or as a snack on their own.

NUTRITION COMPOSITION PER SERVE

Nutrient	Average Qty per serving	%RDI F	M
Energy	782 kj	9%	7%
Protein	2.6 g	5%	4%
Carbohydrate	18 g	8%	6%
Fat	11.8 g	11%	8%
Sodium	30 mg	2%	2%
Fibre	1.2 g	5%	4%

High in omega-3 fats and vitamin E

BAKLAVA CLUSTERS

70 g (¼ packet or 5 sheets) frozen filo pastry, thawed and dried

½ cup (70 g) pistachios, roughly crushed

½ cup (50 g) walnuts, roughly crushed

⅓ cup (50 g) sesame seeds

½ teaspoon ground cinnamon, plus extra for dusting

¼ teaspoon ground cloves

¼ teaspoon ground nutmeg

1 tablespoon raw sugar

SYRUP

½ cup (125 ml) water

½ cup (100 g) raw sugar

Zest 1 lemon

1 tablespoon lemon juice

1 cinnamon stick

3–4 cloves

⅓ cup honey

3 tablespoons extra-virgin olive oil

Preheat the oven to 175°C. Line a 20 x 30 cm lamington tin with baking paper. Layer the filo pastry on the baking paper one at a time and lightly brush each layer with olive oil. Bake for 25 minutes, or until golden brown. Remove from the oven and allow to cool.

Crumble the dried filo pastry into a large bowl, then add the rest of the cluster ingredients and mix well.

To make the syrup, put the water, sugar, lemon zest and juice, cinnamon stick, cloves and honey in a saucepan. Bring to the boil, then reduce the heat and simmer for 5 minutes.

Allow the syrup to cool completely, then whisk in the olive oil. Add the syrup to the cluster mixture and mix well.

Clean the lamington tin and line it with fresh baking paper. Spread the mixture into the tin and bake for 10–15 minutes, or until golden. Remove from the oven, allow to cool completely, then break the mixture into clusters. Store these clusters in an airtight container for up to 2 weeks.

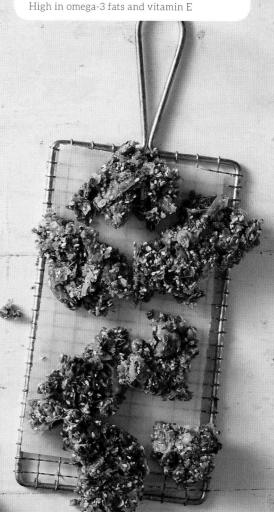

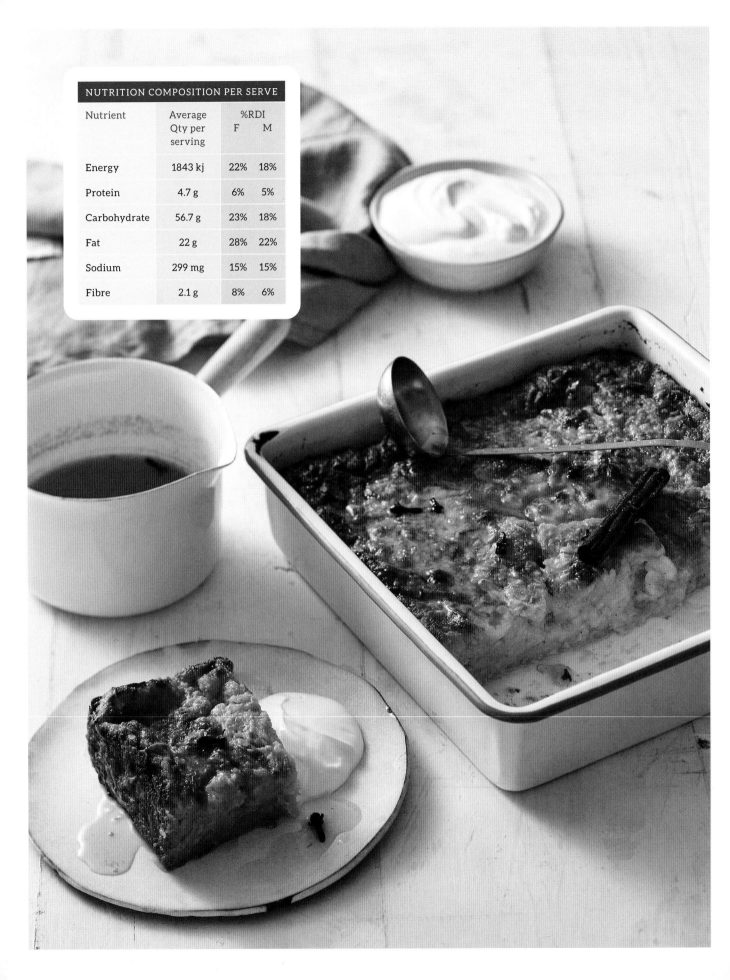

NUTRITION COMPOSITION PER SERVE			
Nutrient	Average Qty per serving	%RDI F	M
Energy	1843 kj	22%	18%
Protein	4.7 g	6%	5%
Carbohydrate	56.7 g	23%	18%
Fat	22 g	28%	22%
Sodium	299 mg	15%	15%
Fibre	2.1 g	8%	6%

Portokalopita:
Greek orange cake

COOKING **45** MINUTES

SERVES **12**

1 cup (250 ml) extra-virgin olive oil,
 plus extra for greasing

375 g frozen filo pastry, thawed

1 ⅓ cups (250 g) golden caster sugar

1 cup (250 g) thick Greek-style yoghurt

Zest 2 oranges

300 ml freshly squeezed orange juice

1 teaspoon vanilla extract

Ground cinnamon

1 tablespoon baking powder

SYRUP

Zest 1 orange

Juice 3 oranges (about 300 ml)

1 cup (200 g) raw sugar

2 cups (500 ml) water

4–5 cloves

1 cinnamon stick

TO SERVE (OPTIONAL)

1 tablespoon thick Greek-style yoghurt

Fresh berries or fruit

Icing sugar, for dusting

Ground cinnamon, for dusting

As I've grown older I've learned that cake is not only for birthdays. Especially this one, which is full of healthy Mediterranean ingredients: extra-virgin olive oil, yoghurt, citrus and aromatic spices.

Preheat the oven to 180°C. Oil the base and sides of a deep 20 x 20 cm cake tin with olive oil. Set your filo pastry out on a clean benchtop so it can dry out while you are making the cake.

Combine all the syrup ingredients in a saucepan over a high heat. Bring to the boil and simmer for 15 minutes. Set aside to cool.

Meanwhile, pour the olive oil into a mixing bowl, add the golden caster sugar and beat with an electric mixer until the mixture is pale and the sugar is completely incorporated. Add the yoghurt, orange zest and juice, vanilla extract and a few pinches of cinnamon, and continue beating until the mixture is smooth. Add the baking powder and mix through.

Tear the filo pastry into small pieces and fold these into the batter before spooning into the oiled tin. Bake for 45 minutes. Pierce the centre of the cake with a skewer; if the skewer comes out clean, the cake is cooked, if not, cook for another few minutes and test again. When the cake is out of the oven, use the skewer to poke holes all over the cake. Pour over the cooled syrup and allow to cool completely.

Slice and serve the cake with the yoghurt, fresh fruit and a dusting of icing sugar and cinnamon, if you like.

Conversion chart

Measuring cups and spoons may vary slightly from one country to another, but the difference is generally not enough to affect a recipe. All cup and spoon measures are level. One Australian metric measuring cup holds 250 ml (8 fl oz), one Australian tablespoon holds 20 ml (4 teaspoons) and one Australian metric teaspoon holds 5 ml. North America, New Zealand and the UK use a 15 ml (3-teaspoon) tablespoon.

LENGTH

Metric	Imperial
3 mm	⅛ inch
6 mm	¼ inch
1 cm	½ inch
2.5 cm	1 inch
5 cm	2 inches
18 cm	7 inches
20 cm	8 inches
23 cm	9 inches
25 cm	10 inches
30 cm	12 inches

LIQUID MEASURES

One American pint	One Imperial pint
500 ml (16 fl oz)	600 ml (20 fl oz)

Cup	Metric	Imperial
⅛ cup	30 ml	1 fl oz
¼ cup	60 ml	2 fl oz
⅓ cup	80 ml	2½ fl oz
½ cup	125 ml	4 fl oz
⅔ cup	160 ml	5 fl oz
¾ cup	180 ml	6 fl oz
1 cup	250 ml	8 fl oz
2 cups	500 ml	16 fl oz
2¼ cups	560 ml	20 fl oz
4 cups	1 litre	32 fl oz

DRY MEASURES

The most accurate way to measure dry ingredients is to weigh them. However, if using a cup, add the ingredient loosely to the cup and level with a knife; don't compact the ingredient unless the recipe requests 'firmly packed'.

Metric	Imperial
15 g	½ oz
30 g	1 oz
60 g	2 oz
125 g	4 oz (¼ lb)
185 g	6 oz
250 g	8 oz (½ lb)
375 g	12 oz (¾ lb)
500 g	16 oz (1 lb)
1 kg	32 oz (2 lb)

OVEN TEMPERATURES

Celsius	Fahrenheit
100°C	200°F
120°C	250°F
150°C	300°F
160°C	325°F
180°C	350°F
200°C	400°F
220°C	425°F

Celsius	Gas mark
110°C	¼
130°C	½
140°C	1
150°C	2
170°C	3
180°C	4
190°C	5
200°C	6
220°C	7
230°C	8
240°C	9
250°C	10

Endnotes

Introduction

7. About 50 people in Australia die each day of heart disease …: Nowbar, A. N., Gitto, M. et al. (2019). 'Mortality from ischemic heart disease: Analysis of data from the world health organization and coronary artery disease risk factors from NCD risk factor collaboration.' *Circulation: Cardiovascular Quality and Outcomes* 12(6); ABC News (2019). 'Heart disease was Australia's leading cause of death in 2018, Australian Bureau of Statistics reveals.' https://www.abc.net.au/news/2019-09-25/heart-disease-australia-leading-cause-death-2018-abs-report/11548358

8. In 1989, American physiologist Ancel Keys and his colleagues …: Keys, A. (1970). 'Coronary heart disease in seven countries: American Heart Association Monograph 29' Circulation 41: 1–211.

8. These trials found that for every point increase …: Dinu, M., Pagliai, G. et al. (2018). 'Mediterranean diet and multiple health outcomes: an umbrella review of meta-analyses of observational studies and randomised trials.' *European Journal of Clinical Nutrition* 72(1): 30–43.

8. A study I conducted with colleagues in Australia …: Itsiopoulos, C., Brazionis, L. et al. (2011). 'Can the Mediterranean diet lower HbA1c in type 2 diabetes? Results from a randomized cross-over study.' *Nutrition, Metabolism & Cardiovascular Disease* 21(9): 740–747.

9. The Mediterranean diet ranked highest in 2018 …: U.S. News Staff (2020). U.S. News 'U.S. News best diets: how we rated 35 eating plans.' https://health.usnews.com/best-diet/best-diets-overall

9. The World Health Organization (WHO) is encouraging a plant-rich diet …: WHO (2018). 'A healthy diet sustainably produced.' Geneva, World Health Organisation.

9. Experts estimate that switching from a Western-style diet …: Saez-Almendros, S., Obrador, B. et al. (2013). 'Environmental footprints of Mediterranean versus Western dietary patterns: beyond the health benefits of the Mediterranean diet.' *Environmental Health: a global access science* source 12: 118.

9. A recently commissioned international collaboration called the EAT-Lancet …: Willett, W. C., Rockstrom, J. et al. (2019). 'Food in the Anthropocene: the EAT–Lancet Commission on healthy diets from sustainable food systems.' *The Lancet* 393(10170): 447–492.

9. In acknowledgement of the impact this diet and lifestyle pattern …: UNESCO (2013). 'Mediterranean diet.' UNESCO https://ich.unesco.org/en/RL/mediterranean-diet-00884

PART ONE: UNDERSTANDING HEART DISEASE AND HOW IT RELATES TO DIET

15. The artery wall is weakened …: Beverly, J. K. and Budoff, M. J. (2020). 'Atherosclerosis: Pathophysiology of insulin resistance, hyperglycemia, hyperlipidemia, and inflammation.' *Journal of Diabetes* 12(2):102–104

16. A comprehensive case control analysis across 52 countries …: Yusuf, S., Hawken, S. et al. (2004). 'Effect of potentially modifiable risk factors associated with myocardial infarction in 52 countries (the INTERHEART study): case-control study.' *The Lancet* 364(9438): 937–952.

19. Diet quality has been directly linked to the risk of developing type 2 diabetes …: Jacobs, S., C. J. Boushey, et al. (2017). 'A priori-defined diet quality indices, biomarkers and risk for type 2 diabetes in five ethnic groups: the Multiethnic Cohort.' *British Journal of Nutrition* 118(4): 312–320.

19. The Mediterranean diet has been demonstrated …: Ryan, M., Itsiopoulos, C. et al. (2013). 'The Mediterranean diet improves hepatic steatosis and insulin sensitivity in individuals with non-alcoholic fatty liver disease.' *Journal of Hepatology*. 59(1): 138–143.

19. Studies have demonstrated that people with a Mediterranean background …: Alcubierre, N., Granado-Casas, M. et al. (2020). 'Spanish people with type 2 diabetes show an improved adherence to the Mediterranean diet.' *Nutrients* 12(2): 560.

20. The most remarkable evidence in support of the cardioprotective effects …: Estruch, R. et al. (2013) 'Primary prevention of cardiovascular disease with a Mediterranean diet.' *New England Journal of Medicine*, 368(14): 1279–1290.

20. It has found that closer adherence to a healthy lifestyle …: Knoops, K. T., de Groot, L. C. et al. (2004). 'Mediterranean diet, lifestyle factors, and 10-year mortality in elderly European men and women: the HALE project.' *JAMA* 292(12): 1433–1439.

20. These results demonstrate that this dietary pattern can be effective …: Williamson, E. J., Polak, J. et al. (2019). 'Sustained adherence to a Mediterranean diet and physical activity on all-cause mortality in the Melbourne Collaborative Cohort Study: application of the g-formula.' *BMC Public Health* 19(1).

21. In that study, about 800 people who had experienced a heart attack …: de Lorgeril M., Salen, P. et al. (1999). 'Mediterranean diet, traditional risk factors, and the rate of cardiovascular complications after myocardial infarction: final report of the Lyon Diet Heart Study.' *Circulation* 99(6): 779–785.

21. However, if the immune system is repeatedly activated …: Bach, E. et al. (2019). 'Systemic, but not local, low-grade endotoxinemia increases plasma sCD163 independently of the cortisol response.' *Endocrine Connections* 8(2): 95–99.

21. Systemic inflammation may be 'inflaming' the brain, vessels, joints and many organs …: Minihane, A. M., Vinoy, S. et al. (2015). 'Low-grade inflammation, diet composition and health: current research evidence and its translation.' *British Journal of Nutrition* 114(7): 999–1012.; Buford, T. W. (2017). '(Dis)Trust your gut: the gut microbiome in age-related inflammation, health, and disease.' *Microbiome* 5(80).

22. These conditions have also been linked to a disturbed gut microbiome.: Cho, I. and Blaser, M. (2012). 'The human microbiome: at the interface of health and disease.' *Nature Reviews Genetics* 13: 260–270.; Buford, T. W. (2017). op. cit.; Bailey, M. A. and Holscher, H. D. (2018). 'Microbiome-mediated effects of the Mediterranean diet on inflammation.' *Advances in Nutrition* 9(3): 193–206.

22. Inflammatory cells release inflammatory chemicals …: Hansson, G. K., Libby, P. et al. (2015). 'Inflammation and plaque vulnerability.' *Journal of Internal Medicine* 278(5): 483–493.

22. In fact, the colon is one of the most densely populated bacterial habitats on Earth.: Sender, R., Fuchs, S. and Milo, R. (2016). 'Revised estimates for the number of human and bacteria cells in the body.' *PLOS Biology* 14(8): e1002533.

22. Fewer beneficial bacteria mean the barrier between the gut …: Brown J. M. and Hazen S. L. (2018). 'Microbial modulation of cardiovascular disease.' *Nature Reviews Microbiology* 16(3). 171–181.

22. Emerging research is pointing to a disturbed or 'dysbiotic' gut microbiome ...: Kouris-Blazos, A. and C. Itsiopoulos (2014). 'Low all-cause mortality despite high cardiovascular risk in elderly Greek-born Australians: attenuating potential of diet?' *Asia Pacific Journal of Clinical Nutrition*. 23(4): 532–544.; Tuohy, K. M., Fava, F. et al. (2014). 'The way to a man's heart is through his gut microbiota: dietary pro and prebiotics for the management of cardiovascular risk.' *Proceedings of the Nutritional Society* 73:172–185.

22. Additionally, gut dysbiosis can also contribute to ...: Virtue A. T., McCright, S. J. et al. (2019). 'The gut microbiota regulates white adipose tissue inflammation and obesity *via a* family of microRNAs'. *Science Translational Medicine* 11 (496): eaav1892

22. A healthy diet rich in plants sustains a healthy gut environment ...: Rothschild, D., Weissbrod, O. et al. (2018). 'Environment dominates over host genetics in shaping human gut microbiota.' *Nature* 555: 210–215.

24. The Lyon Diet Heart Study discussed on ...: de Lorgeril M., et al. (1999). 'Mediterranean diet, traditional risk factors, and the rate of cardiovascular complications after myocardial infarction: final report of the Lion Diet Heart Study.' *Circulation* 99(6): 779–785.

24. Some of these studies have shown that following a Mediterranean diet ...: Schwingshackl, L. and Hoffmann, G. (2014). 'Mediterranean dietary pattern, inflammation and endothelial function: a systematic review and meta-analysis of intervention trials.' *Nutrition, Metabolism & Cardiovascular Disease* 24(9): 929–39.

24. Preliminary results from an ongoing trial in Spain of 1000 people ...: Delgado-Lista, J., P. Perez-Martinez, et al. (2016). 'CORonary Diet Intervention with Olive oil and cardiovascular PREVention study (the CORDIOPREV study): Rationale, methods, and baseline characteristics: A clinical trial comparing the efficacy of a Mediterranean diet rich in olive oil versus a low-fat diet on cardiovascular disease in coronary patients.' *American Heart Journal* 177: 42–50; Gomez-Delgado, F. A., Garcia-Rios, J. F., et al. (2015). 'Chronic consumption of a low-fat diet improves cardiometabolic risk factors according to the CLOCK gene in patients with coronary heart disease.' *Molecular Nutrition & Food Research* 59(12): 2556–2564.

24. This diet also improved vascular function in a sub-group ...: Torres-Peña, J. D., Garcia-Rios, A. et al. (2018). 'Mediterranean diet improves endothelial function in patients with diabetes and prediabetes: A report from the CORDIOPREV study.' *Atherosclerosis* 269: 50–56.

24. Research has shown that an increased polyphenol intake ...: Medina-Remón, A., Casas, A. et al. (2017). 'Polyphenol intake from a Mediterranean diet decreases inflammatory biomarkers related to atherosclerosis: A sub-study of The PREDIMED trial.' *British Journal of Clinical Pharmacology* 83(1):114–128.

24. Evidence suggests that consuming a variety of polyphenols increases ...: Cardona, F., Andrés-Lacueva, C. et al. (2013) 'Benefits of polyphenols on gut microbiota and implications in human health.' *Journal of Nutritional Biochemistry* 24(8): 1415–1422.

24. Extra-virgin olive oil has a higher polyphenol content than refined ...: George, E. S., Marshall, H. L. et al. (2019) 'The effect of high-polyphenol extra virgin olive oil on cardiovascular risk factors: A systematic review and meta-analysis.' *Critical Reviews in Food Science and Nutrition* 59(17): 2772-2795.

24. A Mediterranean diet is also high in omega-3 fatty acids ...: Micallef, M. A., Munro, I. A. and Garg, M. (2009) 'An inverse relationship between plasma n-3 fatty acids and C-reactive protein in healthy individuals.' *European Journal of Clinical Nutrition* 63(9): 1154–1156.

24. Conversely, it also includes very low amounts of processed foods ...: Calder, P. C., Ahluwalia, F. et al. (2011). 'Dietary factors and low-grade inflammation in relation to overweight and obesity.' *British Journal of Nutrition* 106(S3): S1–S78.

25. In the past, a low-fat diet was recommended for people with heart disease ...: Liu A. G., Ford, N. A. et al. (2017). 'A healthy approach to dietary fats: understanding the science and taking action to reduce consumer confusion.' *Nutrition Journal* 16(1): 53–53.

25. Monounsaturated fats help boost HDL 'protective' cholesterol ...: Schwingshackl, L. and Hoffmann, G. (2012). 'Monounsaturated fatty acids and risk of cardiovascular disease: synopsis of the evidence available from systematic reviews and meta-analyses.' *Nutrients* 4(12):1989–2007.

25. Research shows that replacing saturated fats with monounsaturated ...: Liu A. G., Ford, N. A. et al. (2017). op. cit.

25. 'Saturated and trans fats contribute to heart disease ...': Willett, W. C., Stampfer, M. J. et al. (1993). 'Intake of trans fatty acids and risk of coronary heart disease among women.' *The Lancet* 341(8845): 581–585.

25. The Heart Foundation of Australia suggests that people who have type 2 diabetes ...: National Heart Foundation (2020). 'Eggs': https://www.heartfoundation.org.au/healthy-eating/food-and-nutrition/protein-foods/eggs

26. Blood pressure consistently above the normal range ...: National Heart Foundation (2020). 'Blood pressure': https://www.heartfoundation.org.au/your-heart/know-your-risks/blood-pressure.

26. The impact of diet and its components on blood pressure ...: Landowne, M., Thompson, W. and Ruby, B. (1948). 'The minimal sodium diet; a controlled study of its effect upon the blood pressure of ambulatory hypertensive subjects.' *Journal of Laboratory and Clinical Medicine* 33(11): 1482.

26. Since then, several dietary approaches to protect against ...: Appel, L.J. (2017). 'The effects of dietary factors on blood pressure.' *Cardiology Clinics* 35(2): 197–212.

26. Since the 1990s, elevated blood pressure has been acknowledged as a major contributor ...: Kjeldsen, S.E. et al. (2017). 'The Global Burden of Disease Study 2015 and Blood Pressure.' *Blood Pressure* 26(1): 1.

26. Lowering blood pressure levels is associated with reduced ...: Brunstrom, M. and Carlberg, B. (2018). 'Association of blood pressure lowering with mortality and cardiovascular disease across blood pressure levels: a systematic review and meta-analysis.' *JAMA Internal Medicine* 178(1): 28–36.

26. Importantly, life-course studies have shown that ...: Brazionis, L., et al. (2013) 'Diet spanning infancy and toddlerhood is associated with child blood pressure at age 7.5 y.' *American Journal of Clinical Nutrition* 97(6): 1375–86.

26. The most researched of the blood pressure-lowering diets are the DASH ...: Bricarello, P. L., et al. (2018). 'Effects of the Dietary Approach to Stop Hypertension (DASH) diet on blood pressure, overweight and obesity in adolescents: A systematic review.' *Clinical Nutrition ESPEN* 28: 1–11.

26. As illustrated in this section ...: Martinez-Lacoba, R. et al. (2018). 'Mediterranean diet and health outcomes: a systematic meta-review.' *European Journal of Public Health* 28(5): 955–961.

26. A recent review summarising the effects of a Mediterranean diet ...: De Pergola, G. and D'Alessandro, A. (2018). 'Influence of Mediterranean diet on blood pressure.' *Nutrients* 10(11).

26. Among recent studies, adherence to a Mediterranean diet was also associated ...: Lydakis, C. et al. (2012). 'Correlation of blood pressure, obesity, and adherence to the Mediterranean diet with indices of arterial stiffness in children.' *European Journal of Pediatrics* 171(9): 1373–82.

26. In several studies on high-risk individuals ...: Storniolo, C.E. et al. (2017). 'A Mediterranean diet supplemented with extra virgin olive oil or nuts improves endothelial markers involved in blood pressure control in hypertensive women.' *European Journal of Nutrition* 56(1): 89–97.; Davis, C.R. et al. (2017). 'A Mediterranean diet lowers blood pressure and improves endothelial function: results from the MedLey randomized intervention trial.' *American Journal of Clinical Nutrition*. 105(6): 1305–1313.

26. In an Australian study, adults who consumed a Mediterranean diet for 6 months ...: Davis, C.R. et al. (2017). op. cit.

27. This sustained inflammation has also been shown to play a key role ...: Libby P. and Hansson G.K. (2018). 'Taming immune and inflammatory responses to treat atherosclerosis.' *Journal of the American College of Cardiology* 71(2): 173–176.

27. The PREDIMED study found that those following a Mediterranean diet ...: Álvarez-Pérez, J., Sánchez-Villegas, A. et al. (2016). 'Influence of a Mediterranean Dietary Pattern on Body Fat Distribution: Results of the PREDIMED-Canarias Intervention Randomized Trial.' Journal of the American College of Nutrition 35(6):568–580.

27. The Mediterranean diet has consistently proven to be effective ...: Koloverou, E., Esposito, K. et al. (2014). 'The effect of Mediterranean diet on the development of type 2 diabetes mellitus: a meta-analysis of 10 prospective studies and 136,846 participants.' *Metabolism* 63(7): 903–11; Itsiopoulos, C., Brazionis, L. et al. (2011). op. cit.

PART 2: FOLLOWING A MEDITERRANEAN DIET

31. Your brain is a pig ...: Clifton, M. (2019). 'Your brain is a pig: how evolution has primed us to gorge ourselves on fattening foods'. *CBC.ca.* https://www.cbc.ca/life/wellness/your-brain-is-a-pig-how-evolution-has-primed-us-to-gorge-ourselves-on-fattening-foods-1.5082034.

34. There is also a difference in cooking methods and use of ingredients ...: George, E. S., Kucianski, T. et al. (2018). 'A Mediterranean diet model in Australia: strategies for translating the traditional Mediterranean diet into a multicultural setting.' *Nutrients* 10(4).

38. The Heart Foundation recently commissioned an extensive review ...: Collins, C., Burrows, T. et al. (2017) 'Evidence check: Dietary patterns and cardiovascular disease outcomes.' Sax Institute for the National Heart Foundation of Australia. https://www.heartfoundation.org.au/images/uploads/main/For_professionals/Dietary_patterns_and_cardiovascular_disease_outcomes.pdf

38. For people at high risk of heart disease ...: National Heart Foundation (2020). National Heart Foundation, Dietary Position Statement: Heart healthy eating patterns: https://www.heartfoundation.org.au/images/uploads/main/Nutrition_Position_Statement_-_HHEP_v.2.pdf

39. Metabolites produced by beneficial bacteria are important ...: Pastori, D., Carnevale, R. et al. (2017). 'Gut-derived serum lipopolysaccharide is associated with enhanced risk of major adverse cardiovascular events in atrial fibrillation: effect of adherence to Mediterranean diet.' *Journal of the American Heart Association* 6(6).

39. A key benefit of the Mediterranean diet in maintaining a heathy microbiome ...: Del Chierico, F., et. al. (2014). 'Mediterranean diet and health: food effects on gut microbiota and disease control.' *International Journal of Molecular Sciences* 15(7): 11678–11699.

43. It is more nutritious than other legumes ...: Kouris-Blazos, A. and Belski, R. (2016). 'Health benefits of legumes and pulses with a focus on Australian sweet lupins.' *Asia Pacific Journal of Clinical Nutrition* 25(1): 1–17.

43. When embarking on a Mediterranean diet ...: Bailey, M. A. and Holscher, H. D. (2018). op. cit.; Buford, T. W. (2017). op. cit.

46. An analysis of average weekly food costs in a study ...: Opie, R. S., Segal, L. et al. (2015). 'Assessing healthy diet affordability in a cohort with major depressive disorders.' *Journal of Public Health and Epidemiology* 7(5): 159–169.

46. Remarkably, the people following the Mediterranean-style eating pattern ...: Jacka, F. N., O'Neil, A. et al. (2018) A randomised controlled trial of dietary improvement for adults with major depression (the 'SMILES' trial).' *BMC Medicine* 16: 236.

48. The healthy immigrant effect (HIE) ...: Kennedy, S., et. al. (2015). 'The healthy immigrant effect: patterns and evidence from four countries.' *Journal of International Migration and Integration* 16(2): 317–332.

48. However, over time, after increasing years of living in their new country ...: Satia-Abouta, J. (2003). 'Dietary Acculturation: Definition, Process, Assessment and Implications.' *International Journal of Human Ecology* 4(1).

48. We understand that this resistance to change ...: Anikeeva, O., et al. (2010). 'Review paper: the health status of migrants in Australia: a review.' *Asia Pacific Journal of Public Health* 22(2): 159–193.

48. Other produce commonly grown by our study subjects ...: Thodis, A. (2019). 'MEDiterranean ISlands – Australia Study: Greek Mediterranean diet pattern adherence, successful aging and associations in Greek Australian island-born long-term migrants.' La Trobe University, Melbourne, Australia.

48. Maintaining a fruit and vegetable garden ...: Radd-Vagenas, S., Kouris-Blazos, A. et al. (2016) 'Evolution of Mediterranean Diets and Cuisine: Concepts and Definitions.' *Asia Pacific Journal of Clinical Nutrition* 26(5): 749–763.

48. As well as increasing physical activity and improving vitamin D status ...: Morgan, G., Rocha, C. and Poynting, S. (2005). 'Grafting cultures: longing and belonging in immigrants' gardens and backyards in Fairfield.' *Journal of Intercultural Studies* 26(1): 93–105.

48. Few studies have investigated the role of backyard fruit and vegetable gardens ...: Pillen H., Tsourtos, G. et al. (2017). 'Retaining traditional dietary practices among Greek immigrants to Australia: the role of ethnic identity.' *Ecology of Food and Nutrition* 56(4): 312–328.

PART 3: YOUR HEART HEALTH TOOLKIT

57. We've gone for options that maintain the nutritional benefits ...: Burlingame, B. and Dernini, S. (2011). 'Sustainable diets: The Mediterranean diet as an example.' *Public Health and Nutrition* 14: 2285–2287.

xx. 'We've gone for options that maintain the nutritional benefits ...': Burlingame, B. and S. Dernini, (2011). op cit.

About Dr Catherine Itsiopoulos

Dr Catherine Itsiopoulos (PhD APD) is Pro Vice Chancellor College of Science, Health, Engineering and Education and a Professor of Nutrition and Dietetics at Murdoch University. An Accredited Practising Dietitian and a recognised expert in Nutrition and Dietetics, Catherine has international standing as a leader in Mediterranean diet research. She is the inaugural chair of the international scientific advisory committee of the Olive Wellness Institute and is on the scientific advisory committee of the International Nut and Dried Fruit Council. She has a particular interest in the Mediterranean diet, and she is the lead investigator of the AUSMED Heart Trial focused on secondary prevention of heart disease with a Mediterranean diet.

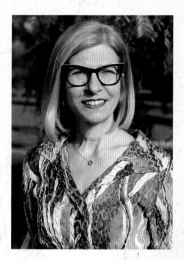

Catherine has spent almost 30 years investigating the health benefits of the traditional Greek (Cretan) Mediterranean diet cuisine on prevention and management of diseases that are linked to poor diet and lifestyle. She has authored over 100 scientific publications on the findings of this cardioprotective diet, presented her research nationally and internationally, and has published two cookbooks on the Mediterranean diet: *The Mediterranean Diet* (2013) and *The Mediterranean Diet Cookbook* (2015).

About the contributors

Associate Professor Colleen Thomas leads the Cardiovascular Physiology Laboratory at La Trobe University. She has researched expertise and international standing as a translational cardiovascular physiologist. She is a recognised leader in coronary heart disease research — particularly in the areas of developing novel drugs and strategies to treat heart attacks. Functional components of Mediterranean diet to prevent or reverse chronic cardiovascular disease and diabetes is also a significant focus of her clinical work. She also investigates gut microbial involvement in cardiovascular disease pathogenesis.

Dr Hannah Mayr is an Accredited Practicing Dietitian. Her PhD at La Trobe University investigated the effects of a Mediterranean diet on inflammation and adiposity in people with coronary heart disease. Hannah is a research dietitian at Princess Alexandra Hospital, where she is involved in implementing evidence for the Mediterranean diet into routine care for people with chronic diseases. Hannah is also involved in research capacity building for clinical dietitians, and is a lecturer in the Bond University Master of Nutrition and Dietetic Practice.

Dr Jane Willcox is a senior lecturer and research dietician at the School of Allied Health, Human Services and Sport at La Trobe University. She is also an honorary Research Fellow with the University of Auckland. Jane has worked for more than 20 years in clinical dietetics and public health, including at The Alfred in heart and lung transplant and cardiology, and at The Baker Heart and Diabetes Institute (International Diabetes Institute). Her interests include nutrition interventions and communication with a focus on disease prevention.

Associate Professor Andrew Wilson is on the Department of Cardiology and the University Department of Medicine at St Vincent's Hospital in Melbourne and the St Vincent's Institute. He is also the director of the University of Melbourne's Lipid and Cardiovascular Risk Reduction Clinic, and an NHF DART Clinical Research Fellow. His clinical interests are in all areas of Interventional Cardiology and Assessment and Therapy of Cardiovascular Risk, particularly in high-risk patients such as those with insulin resistance, renal disease and peripheral arterial disease. Andrew spent three years working at Stanford Medical Center in California, and he now leads the Translational Cardiovascular Biology group and is involved in a range of projects focused on biomarkers of atherosclerosis and links between insulin resistance and cardiovascular disease.

Associate Professor Antigone Kouris has more than 30 years' experience as a dietitian clinician in private practice. She is a researcher on the Mediterranean diet, and has authored over 50 published papers, co-authored seven university textbooks and written three of her own books, including a Mediterranean diet cookbook. She has also worked as a food-product developer using legumes (lupins). Her pioneering PhD was the first study to show in the 1990s that adherence to a Mediterranean diet pattern (MDP) in old age conferred longevity. She holds an adjunct position at La Trobe university teaching dietetics and conducting research on her lupin cookies (skinnybik.com).

Dr Antonia Thodis is an Accredited Practising Dietitian with clinical and research experience in delivering nutrition counselling and interventions for cancer care, cardiovascular health and supporting cognitive function among elderly, migrant and CALD populations. Her research area of interest is the traditional Mediterranean diet and dietary pattern evolved from past Australian migrant studies and in part, her Greek heritage. Her PhD research – the Mediterranean Islands (MEDIS) Australia study was completed at La Trobe University in 2019.

Dr Elena George is an Accredited Practising Dietitian and Lecturer in Nutrition and Dietetics at Deakin University. Elena's parents and grandparents migrated from Greece and Cyprus, and they imparted a passion for Mediterranean food and lifestyle. Her heritage and love of good food has instilled in her a desire to enhance evidence-based practice in dietetics through research. A particular area of interest is in the development and delivery of dietary interventions (Mediterranean diet) for the prevention and management of chronic diseases. She is particularly interested in translating traditional dietary patterns in Western and multicultural populations.

Associate Professor Laima Brazionis is a research nutritionist, nutritional epidemiologist and PhD supervisor at La Trobe University. She is a University of Melbourne graduate in optometry and ocular therapeutics, and her early Mediterranean diet studies contributed to her Master of Human Nutrition (Deakin University) and PhD (Medicine, Monash University). Her current role as an Academic Specialist in the Department of Medicine (University of Melbourne) involves collaborations with cardiologists, endocrinologists, basic scientists, indigenous researchers and a telemedicine technology team. She is also a Chief Investigator in a Centre of Research Excellence (NHMRC) at the Clinical Trials Centre (University of Sydney).

Dr Marno Ryan is a gastroenterologist based at St Vincent's Hospital in Melbourne, where she is involved in research into hepatic metabolism of fats and carbohydrates, with a focus on dietary interventions. She specialises in hepatology, with a particular interest in fatty liver and viral hepatitis. She completed her advanced training at St Vincent's Hospital Melbourne before undertaking an MD investigating the relationship between non-alcoholic fatty liver disease (NAFLD) and features of the Metabolic Syndrome. She then spent two years working at the laboratory of Professor Gerald Reaven at Stanford University, California.

Teagan Kucianski is an Accredited Practicing Dietitian, Pharmacist and Lecturer in Nutrition and Dietetics at Latrobe University. She is currently completing her PhD in the area of the Mediterranean diet and heart disease. Teagan has worked as a dietitian as well as pharmacist, and her research interests include translating the Mediterranean diet for multicultural populations, the Mediterranean diet in cardiovascular disease and the development of questionnaires suitable for assessing Mediterranean diet adherence in multicultural populations such as Australia.

Acknowledgements

The Heart Health Guide is my third book on the Mediterranean diet, and I could not have produced this book without the support of my loving family, dear friends, research colleagues and the Pan Macmillan team.

Hippocrates from the Greek Island of Kos (460–370 BC) was a Greek physician often referred to as the 'Father of Medicine', and he coined the phrase 'Let food be thy medicine and medicine be thy food'. It was as though he was speaking directly to the health benefits of the Mediterranean diet. Growing up in a Greek Mediterranean family in the northern suburbs of Melbourne, I was used to the Greek traditions of home-cooked meals where vegetables from my father Thanasi's large backyard garden were the hero of the meal. My mother would prepare the tastiest vegetable-based casseroles like fassoulakia yiaxni made with a fresh tomato purée (called saltsa) that we prepared in the backyard. Each autumn the whole extended family would get together and prepare the saltsa from ripe fresh tomatoes with the help from our Italian neighbours who had specialised equipment imported from Italy. There was always plenty of vegetables and saltsa to share with neighbours!

My career as a clinical dietitian and nutrition researcher has brought together my love of food and science, desire to work with people to improve their health, and a spirit of discovery. I was privileged to meet a wonderful mentor early in my career, Prof. Kerin O'Dea AO, who researches the therapeutic effects of traditional hunter-gatherer diets. She inspired me to look beyond nutrients and focus on healthy eating patterns, and has mentored and supported my research career.

I have the AUSMED Heart Trial collaborators to thank for their phenomenal commitment to the multicentre trial that investigates the impact of the traditional Greek Mediterranean diet on secondary prevention of heart disease. I sincerely thank Prof. Kerin O'Dea and Prof. Peter Brooks who brought me together with the team of cardiologists Prof. Andrew Wilson and Prof. William van Gaal, gastroenterologist Dr Marno Ryan, and nutritional epidemiologist Assoc. Prof. Laima Brazionis to conceptualise the AUSMED Heart Trial. We were then joined by cardiovascular physiologist Assoc. Prof. Colleen Thomas, exercise physiologist Prof. Michael Kingsley, cardiologist Prof. Miguel Ángel Martínez-González, epidemiologist Dr Hassan Vally, health economist Prof. Leonie Segal, dietitians Assoc. Prof. Antigone Kouris-Blazos, Dr Audrey Tierney and Dr Jane Willcox, biostatistician Assoc. Prof. Agus Salim, dietetic PhD students and graduates Teagan Kucianski, Dr Antonia Thodis, Dr Elena George, and most importantly Dr Hannah Mayr, who led the AUSMED Heart Trial Pilot study for her doctoral studies.

I would like to thank the Pan Macmillan team for making this book possible. I sincerely thank Ingrid Ohlsson for her inspiration in conceptualising the heart health focus of this book, and for her support and mentorship throughout the project. I thank Naomi van Groll for her project management and Katie Bosher and Danielle Walker for their meticulous recipe and content editing and for keeping me on track. For the fabulous look of this book I owe thanks to the designer Madeleine Kane, photographer Rob Palmer, stylist Emma Knowles and home economist Kerrie Ray.

I owe my successful career to my amazing family. My late father Thanasi who inspired me and my sister to get a university education, which he said was our 'ticket to a successful life', my mother Theano who is a wonderful cook and food critic and passed on her special family recipes, and my dear sister Anna who persevered in capturing the family recipe details. Without my loving husband and soulmate Savvas Koutsis, I could not have achieved a great balance between family and career. Savvas was there by my side from the early 80s when he'd drive me over 100 kilometres to Deakin Uni in Geelong to do experiments on how to prevent tomato paste moulds, to the current day where he is my greatest supporter and reminds me to never doubt myself and to go for it!

A final heartfelt thank you to my precious daughters Tiana and Vivienne who were babies when I started my PhD and have helped me produce the cookbooks. Many of the recipes are inspired by my girls, especially the vegetarian ones. Now they're young adults and have just moved out of the family home to start their lives on their own. As they both love to cook and entertain we made sure they had a fully equipped kitchen stocked with all the ingredients to continue the Mediterranean way of life (and an open door to come home anytime and have Mamma and Yiayias' cooking).

Index

First published 2020 in Macmillan
by Pan Macmillan Australia Pty Limited
Level 25, 1 Market Street, Sydney,
New South Wales, Australia 2000

A CIP catalogue record for this book is available from the National Library of Australia:
http://catalogue.nla.gov.au

Design and illustrations by Madeleine Kane
Edited by Katie Bosher
Index by Helena Holmgren
Prop and food styling by Emma Knowles
Food preparation by Kerrie Ray
Colour + reproduction by Splitting Image Colour Studio
Printed in China by Imago Printing International Limited

Image on page 6 © Unsplash; images on page 12 © Unsplash, Stocksy, iStock; image on page
15 © Unsplash; images on page 23 © Shutterstock; images on page 28 © Unsplash, iStock;
image on page 30 © Stocksy; image on page 35 © iStock; image on page 42 © iStock; image
on page 44-45 © Shutterstock; image on page 49 © iStock; images on page 50 © Unsplash,
Stocksy, iStock; image on page 52 © iStock; image on page 59 © iStock; image on page
65 © iStock; images on page 74 © Unsplash, iStock; image on page 88 © Stocksy.

Diagram on page 23 © 2017 TW Buford; Australian Dietary Guidelines on page 37 ©
Commonwealth of Australia 2016; diagram on page 41 © Dr Hannah Mayr; diagram
on page 57 © 2018 B. Burlingame and S. Dernini; diagram on page 62 © 2010 Fundacion
Dieta Mediterranea; diagram on page 64 © Commonwealth of Australia 2016.

10 9 8 7 6 5 4 3 2 1